MALE SEXUAL HEALTH

MALE SEXUAL HEALTH

Philip R. Roen, M.D., F.A.C.S.

WILLIAM MORROW & COMPANY, INC.
NEW YORK, 1974

Illustrations by Charles Stern

DESIGN BY HELEN ROBERTS

PRINTED IN THE UNITED STATES OF AMERICA.

2 3 4 5

Library of Congress Cataloging in Publication Data

Roen, Philip R
Male sexual health.

1. Generative organs, Male–Diseases. I. Title.
[DNLM: 1. Health education. 2. Prostatic diseases –Popular works. 3. Urologic diseases–Popular works.
WJ752 R715m 1973]
RC875.R65 1974 616.6 73-14854
ISBN 0-688-00223-4

To the memory of Neil

Acknowledgments

Much praise to my editor, Eunice Riedel, whose advice was invaluable. Many, many thanks to my secretary, Maryann Worsnop, for all of her work on the manuscript.

Contents

List of Illustrations

Introduction

> "I am worried sick. I went to see my doctor because I thought I had some sort of bladder trouble and also because I haven't been too good sexually lately, and my doctor sent me to you, a specialist. He thinks I have a prostate condition. I thought only older men got prostate trouble—I'm only thirty-four. Am I old before my time?"

Most of my patients, no matter how well educated they are, know surprisingly little about their sexual apparatus.

Our society places excessive emphasis on the outward signs of maleness—including such nonsense as the size of a man's penis. But the internal structures that truly control a man's sexual life, and which determine so much of his health and happiness, are little-known and surrounded with misinformation or old wives' tales.

Impotence in particular is almost always treated as a joke in public, even though it's a rare man who will never have to confront it. Ignorance of its causes and of treatment possibilities has led to a tremendous amount of unnecessary suffering. And the prostate —central to so many male maladies—is something most men know they have, but many would be hard put to say exactly where it is, what it does, and what danger signals to watch for.

Often men—like my patient above—believe that they needn't worry about their prostates until they get older. And, of course, it is true that prostate and other male urogenital problems tend to be most common in older men. But plenty of men in their twenties to forties also develop these ailments. Indeed, teen-agers, young boys, and even newborn babies can have medical problems associated with the prostate. Even women aren't immune, for women sometimes have urinary symptoms connected with what we call the "female prostate."

And people need to know the facts, for prostate trouble is widespread. About one man in three over the age of fifty will develop some kind of prostatic problem, and almost half of these men will require surgery. Prostatic cancer is the third leading cause of cancer deaths in men over fifty-five—only cancers of the lung and the lower intestine kill more men. Yet many men—unaware that this disease usually causes no symptoms until it is too late for a cure—

still do not realize how vital it is to have their prostates checked regularly by a doctor.

Even the more common enlargements and inflammations, which could often be so easily treated, are allowed to worsen because men don't realize the seriousness of urinating too frequently, feebly, slowly, or incompletely. Assuming that urinary problems are unimportant or simply a sign of growing older, men too often wait until alarming symptoms develop before going to the doctor.

Not only with impotence and prostate trouble, but also just about every other area of male sexual health, myths have filled the vacuum left by lack of correct information. Some men have strange ideas that vasectomy would make them impotent—even that it is the same as castration. Many believe that older men should have no need for sex. And almost everyone seems to be confused about male sex hormones, "male menopause," whether surgery on the urogenital tract will leave a man sterile or impotent, and many other questions whose answers could relieve fear and protect health.

The aim of this book is to dispel the mystery that envelops the male sexual and urinary tracts. I will explain what ailments can arise, what symptoms to watch for, and what treatment is called for.

Though I am writing almost exclusively about men, I hope that this book will also be read by women, so that they will better understand the maladies that might afflict the men they love.

MALE SEXUAL HEALTH

1. The Prostate, Testicles, and Penis

> "My boss is in the hospital with prostate trouble and he has all sorts of tubes in him. Frankly, I don't even know *what* the prostate is or *where* it is."

For those of you who, like the man above, are a bit foggy about male anatomy, I am going to present this complex and intricate mechanism in simple form.

THE PROSTATE

The prostate is the most important of the internal sex organs. On its healthy functioning depend both a man's sexual activity and his urinary flow.

Where is the prostate?

The prostate is located at the exit of the bladder. Running through it is the urethra, the tube which carries urine from the bladder to the tip of the penis. The prostate almost completely encircles the urethra as it joins the bladder.

Also encased in the prostate are two ejaculatory ducts, which receive the sperm from the testicles via the seminal vesicles. The seminal vesicles—tubular structures which supply secretions to nourish the sperm—are found behind the bladder close to its exit but higher than the prostate.

How large is it?

At birth, the prostate is smaller than a grain of rice. Though it becomes larger as a boy grows older, it begins significant growth only at puberty, when it is stimulated by male sex hormone. In a grown man, it reaches the size of a large chestnut. If it starts to grow abnormally, as we shall see later, it can enlarge immensely, sometimes to the size of a baseball or even larger.

Why is it so important to have a doctor check your prostate?

Because the prostate sits between the bladder and the rectum, it can be felt by a physician who inserts his finger through the anus (the rectal exit). Though

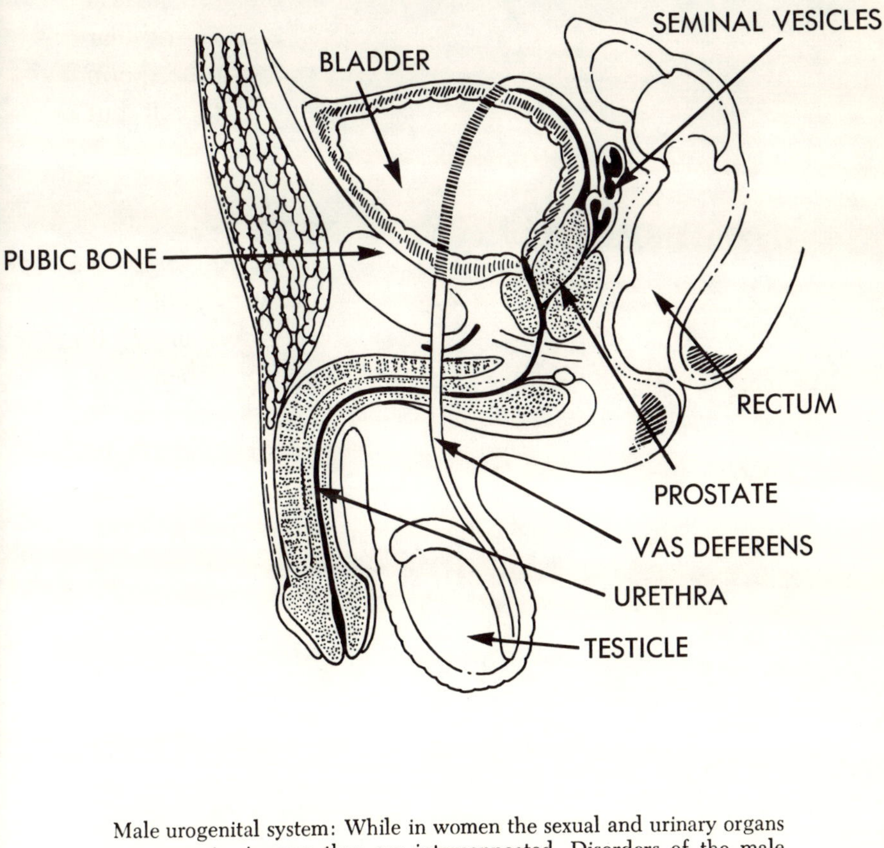

Male urogenital system: While in women the sexual and urinary organs are separate, in men they are interconnected. Disorders of the male urogenital tract can therefore cause both urinary and sexual problems.

many men find this examination embarrassing or disagreeable, it should never be left out of a man's checkup. The doctor's finger in the rectum can tell him about many ailments—from a simple infection to cancer—not only of the prostate but of the rectal and anal area as well.

Why is a healthy prostate sexually important?

The prostate is made up partly of muscle fibers and partly of glandular cells which produce a secretion or fluid. This fluid is manufactured constantly—about five to thirty drops every hour, and much larger amounts during sexual excitement. Some of the fluid normally and continuously seeps down through many tiny collecting ducts, to lubricate the urethra. The rest remains in the prostate.

When a man has an ejaculation—with intercourse, or masturbation, or even in a wet dream during sleep—the muscles of the prostate contract and force the stored fluid out into the urethra; here it mixes with sperm cells and with secretions from the seminal vesicles. Serving as a medium in which the sperm swim, the prostatic fluid is the major part of the ejaculate—which can vary from half a thimbleful to as much as a tablespoonful.

Why are prostate trouble and urinary problems so often connected?

Because the prostate, the seminal vesicles, and the ejaculatory ducts lie so close to the bladder and urethra, any urinary difficulty may spread to them, and disorders of the prostate may affect the urinary tract. For example, since the prostate surrounds the urethra, any enlargement of the prostate can compress that tube, making it very difficult or even impossible to pass urine.

Urination can sometimes be affected because of the nearness of the prostate gland to the two urinary control muscles, or sphincters. These surround the urethra, one just above, the other just below the prostate. If these control muscles, or the nerves to these muscles, are damaged, a man can have little or no urinary control. This distressing condition has a number of other causes, such as nerve diseases that diminish the sphincter action, but the most common cause is damage to the control muscles during prostatic surgery.

Similarly, if nerve damage should occur during a prostatic operation, impotence may result.

THE TESTICLES

What do the testicles do?

The testicles—the two egg-shaped organs in the scrotum, the sac that hangs between the upper thighs—are double factories: they make sperm cells and male sex hormones, including testosterone.

How big should they be?

Their size varies—from that of pigeon's eggs to that of hen's eggs.

How do sperm cells get from the testicles to the penis?

In its position "outside" the body, the testicle is connected by a cord, about the thickness of a lead pencil, which contains blood vessels, nerves, and a tube called the vas deferens. It is this tube which carries the sperm to the ejaculatory ducts in the urethra, which runs the length of the penis.

Sperm cells are formed from microscopic structures in the testicles and are collected in fine tubules. The tiny tubules unite into one larger tube which coils intricately at the back of the testicle to form a structure called the epididymis. This coiled epididymis stores the sperm cells until they migrate or are propelled through the vas deferens to the urethra, where they join with secretions from the prostate and seminal vesicles to form the semen.

How many sperm cells does a man produce?

In many animals and birds, the testicles do not make sperm cells during most of the year. Only during the autumn breeding season do they burst into activity, insuring that conception will take place then and that the young will be born in the spring, the most favorable time for growth and development. But men produce sperm throughout the year. Even though only one sperm cell is necessary to fertilize the female egg, a man produces sperm in astronomical numbers; on an average, about fifteen drops of ejaculation fluid contain more than 60 million sperm. During his lifetime, a man may produce about 400 billion sperm cells.

How are the male sex hormones made?

The male hormones, or androgens, including testosterone, are manufactured in many small cell nests embedded among the sperm tubules in the testicles. Unlike sperm, which follow a limited path through the body to be ejaculated through the penis, the hormones go directly into the blood and reach all parts of the body.

Is it only the testicles that make a man's sex hormones?

Some androgens are made elsewhere in the body (in the adrenal gland, for example), but only the testicles produce testosterone. Although other androgens are necessary for life while testosterone is not, testosterone is most important sexually because without it the changes of puberty cannot occur. Other androgens can compensate only partly for lack of testosterone.

How does puberty happen?

A child's testicles probably function little, if at all, until they are triggered by hormones from the pituitary gland, located at the base of the skull. This usually happens when a boy is between eleven and fourteen, though some boys mature earlier or later. At this point, the testicles begin to produce testosterone, which starts the changes we associate with puberty.

Male sex hormone causes some obvious physical alterations: the boy's voice becomes deeper; his penis and scrotum enlarge; hair grows on his pubic area, underarms, and face; his skin becomes oilier (sometimes he develops acne); and he is apt to have a sudden spurt of growth. About half of all boys have enlarged and tender breasts, but only temporarily. Within the boy's body, less visible changes occur: the accessory sex glands (such as the prostate and seminal vesicles) begin to enlarge and increase their secretions. Finally, as any parent of an adolescent knows, there are psychological changes—the boy is apt to be moody, aggressive, and full of conflicts. These physical and emotional changes are normal characteristics of puberty and are brought about by testosterone production.

What if something is wrong with his testicles?

When the testicles do not function because of illness (mumps, for example) or because they have been injured or removed *before* puberty, a boy will become a eunuch. His penis remains small, his prostate and seminal vesicles fail to mature, no sperm is produced, and the normal secondary sex characteristics never appear—he grows no facial hair and his voice does not deepen. Instead, the long bones of his arms and legs lengthen—too much in proportion to his trunk—and he will have a tendency to fat in places where a girl normally forms it, such as at the hips. Such a man is of course sterile, sexual feeling is nonexistent, and he is usually incapable of having either an erection or an ejaculation.

Boys who produce little or no testosterone can be treated with artificial testosterone given by injection (oral medication is less effective) at intervals, which will bring on all of the normal pubertal changes; however, artificial hormones will, of course, not make these boys fertile.

What happens if the testicles are lost after puberty?

In this case female characteristics do not replace male ones. These men retain their deep voices, facial and pubic hair, and normal internal sex organs. In fact, many adult men who have been castrated surgically can still have intercourse. This happens because the testicles have functioned long enough to have produced normal male development and sexual habits. But, of course, these men are sterile, because only the testicles can produce sperm cells. And unless one gives them hormone injections, their penises will shrink somewhat.

Thus testosterone administered by injection (or in tablet form) can substitute for natural production when this is inadequate.

However, the testicles are sometimes removed in cases of cancer of the prostate in order to eliminate the hormone, as testosterone stimulates this type of cancer. In such cases, the hormone would of course not be replaced.

Is testosterone a factor in homosexuality?

No. Male homosexuals have normal testosterone production, as well as normal penises and internal sexual organs; they are capable of erection and ejaculation, have essentially normal sperm production, and are fertile. Their preferred sexual activities are in almost all cases psychologically induced.

What could keep a man from producing sperm?

A man's ability to make sperm cells is of course permanently destroyed by castration, and it can be reduced in several other ways, such as by exposure to X rays or radioactivity, by alcoholism, or by vitamin B_1 deficiency.

We have good evidence of what radioactivity can do from excellent studies on the survivors of Hiroshima. Depending upon how much radioactivity they were exposed to, they became either temporarily or permanently sterile. In some cases of temporary sterility, their children were born deformed. Because of this known damage by X ray and radioactivity, physicians are often careful to protect a child's or young man's testicles with a lead shield when the lower abdomen must be X-rayed. However, any minor damage caused by such X-ray exposure is temporary.

Similarly, sperm counts are low in alcoholics and in cases of starvation or nutritional deficiency. All of these instances probably have a common cause—low vitamin

B_1 intake, which has an indirect action on testicular function via the pituitary gland. Attempts to restore sperm production must be made by vitamin B_1 injections in very large amounts. Taking vitamin pills is insufficient for alcoholics, who generally have liver damage which interferes with oral absorption and body use of many necessary food factors.

In rats, vitamin E is necessary for adequate sperm production and its lack prevents normal testicular function. However, since vitamin E is present in so many common foods, vitamin E deficiency does not ordinarily occur in men who eat a normal varied diet; taking vitamin E capsules is therefore unnecessary.

Isn't the temperature of the testicles important for sperm production?

Yes. Because of their location outside the body, the temperature of the testicles is lower by a few degrees than the normal body temperature; and this is quite important for reproduction. In experiments with animals in which the scrotum was wrapped in insulating material so that its temperature rose, the animals soon became sterile; when the insulation was removed, so that the scrotal temperature dropped, the animals again became fertile. In many mammals, the testicles are high and not in the scrotum during most of the year. During this period the animals are not fertile; only during the short breeding season, when the testicles descend into the scrotum temporarily, can they reproduce.

In like fashion, when a testicle does not descend

into the scrotum in a man (as a result of a birth deficiency) but remains in the abdomen, it is subject to the slightly higher body temperature and will not make sperm cells.

Don't such testicles usually descend as a boy grows?

Although in about 4 percent of boys under sixteen either one or both testicles have not descended, in the vast majority of cases (more than three-quarters) they will descend spontaneously at or before puberty. Nevertheless, slowly progressive degenerative changes begin in a nondescended testicle at about age five, and the testicle will probably not grow normally even if it does descend spontaneously at around puberty.

What should be done about undescended testicles?

It is best to operate on the undescended testicle to bring it down into the scrotum when the patient is between the ages of five and seven. I have operated upon many children beyond this age (but before puberty) for this problem and have found to my dismay and theirs that follow-up study years after the operation shows them to be infertile. An operation for an undescended testicle at any time beyond puberty is worthless for preserving sperm production. Thus, the earlier the descent—either natural or surgical—the greater the likelihood of normal development; without doubt, the scrotal sac is an effective thermal regulator essential to normal testicular function. An even more urgent reason for securing descent of the testicle is that there have been twenty-two times as many cases of cancer in undescended testicles as in normal testicles in the scrotum.

Can a fever cause sterility?

A severe illness with long-continued fever may cause the testicles to suffer as a result of high temperature, but usually the loss of function is only temporary.

What about trying birth control by raising the scrotal temperature (with hot baths, for example)?

This is not effective in practice: the Scandinavians with their frequent, very high-temperature sauna baths and the Japanese with their equally scalding hot baths have normal fertility rates.

THE PENIS

The penis is composed basically of elastic, loose skin covering three tubes. One of these, the urethra, conducts urine from the bladder and also serves as a passageway for the ejaculate at sexual climax. The other two long tubes, called corpora cavernosa, are spongelike structures which enable the penis to become rigid or erect. These corpora are made up of thousands

What are "wet dreams"?

Wet dreams or nocturnal emissions are natural ways for the body to get rid of accumulated sperm and secretions when a man has not ejaculated for some time either with coitus or masturbation. This kind of emission can occur without sexual fantasy in dreams and can happen at any age—in a boy just beyond puberty with awakening sex activity, in a sexually abstinent man (such as a priest), or in a man deprived of sex for a prolonged period (such as a prisoner). It is a natural outlet and is not a sign of illness, abnormality, or "bad thoughts."

What about circumcision?

Most physicians, myself included, feel that baby boys should be circumcised routinely at birth unless there is a specific medical reason against it. In later life, an uncircumcised man is more apt to have problems such as infections under the hood of skin, or inability to retract the foreskin, or even cancer of the penis, than a man who is circumcised.

An accumulation of smegma (the material secreted by tiny glands under the foreskin) tends to irritate, particularly when the foreskin cannot be pulled back to permit proper cleansing; with prolonged skin irritation, cancer of the penis may form directly under the foreskin.

Among Jewish people, who practice circumcision at

birth, cancer of the penis is unknown. Among Mohammedans, who practice circumcision at puberty, cancer of the penis is rare but does occur. In uncircumcised men, cancer of the penis accounts for about 1 percent of all malignant growths.

Even if it were not for the serious cancer potentiality, I believe every male child should be circumcised very early in life for the sake of cleanliness alone.

2. Inflammations of the Prostate

> A young man studying in a Roman Catholic seminary visited my office and said he had the "priest's disease." He had been able to diagnose his own case, he said, because it was common scuttlebutt among the priesthood that absence of regular sexual activity would often produce prostate trouble and cause frequency of urination, backache, and discomfort on voiding.
>
> Was this twenty-three-year-old seminarian correct? Did he have prostate trouble, and had he diagnosed his own problem?
>
> You bet he had!

Actually, the prostate gland develops two kinds of inflammation. One is a true infection, caused by bacteria. The other, which we call a "congested prostate" or prostatitis, involves no infection even though it causes almost the same symptoms. Because these inflammations are different in origin, we treat each somewhat differently.

How does your doctor know which kind of inflammation you have?

When we suspect prostatitis, we first examine the prostate gland by inserting a gloved finger into the rectum to determine the *size* of the gland, whether it is *smooth* or nodular (the latter often denotes cancer or stones), and whether it is of normal *consistency* or firmness, too soft or too hard (another sign of cancer). Most important, we squeeze some fluid out of the prostate to study under the microscope.

Why must a doctor examine the prostatic fluid?

Even if the prostate seems entirely normal to the touch, there may be pus cells and bacteria which only the microscope can reveal. If there is no pus, we take some of the prostatic fluid for culture—that is, we place it in a test tube with suitable "food" or growth material so that any bacteria present in the fluid yet not easily seen microscopically will increase in number. Laboratory study can then identify the particular germ.

Often no germs are present, and then the physician will rule out infectious prostatitis and look for further clues to the congestive type.

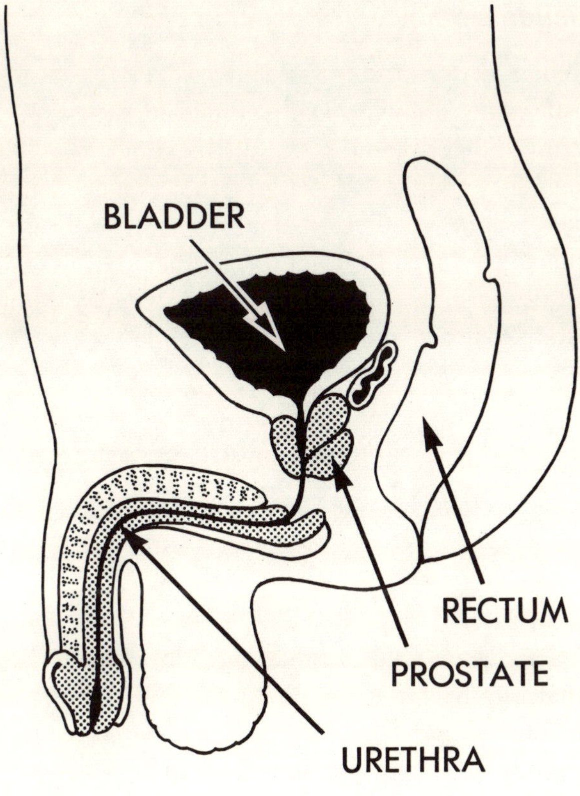

How the prostate causes urinary symptoms: Because the prostate encircles the urethra where it leaves the bladder, prostate problems often cause urinary symptoms.

CONGESTIVE PROSTATITIS

What makes a congested prostate inflamed if there aren't any germs?

You will remember that the prostate is composed of many tiny secreting glands surrounded by muscle fibers, and that when these muscles contract in ejaculation, they squeeze the glands and empty them. But what happens if a man does not ejaculate? Well, then the fluid within these glands stagnates—it begins to decompose, and many cast-off cells and other materials accumulate. All of this results in the inflammation we call congestive prostatitis.

Prostatitis in a young man is therefore frequently the result of poor sexual practices. Any male who abstains totally from masturbation or intercourse, and thus fails to empty his prostate periodically, risks developing the "priest's disease."

Is abstinence the only cause of prostatitis?

No. Paradoxically, the other extreme—either excessive masturbation, excessive intercourse, or prolongation of sexual excitement—can cause exactly the same condition. Although a single episode will not harm the prostate, repeated insults over a considerable period of time may.

One of my patients, a sixty-two-year-old bachelor who had for some twenty years required occasional treatment for mild prostatitis, persuaded a woman in her late twenties to live with him. He was now called upon to satisfy her sexual appetite by trying to have coitus almost daily, though his own sexual needs would have been answered by intercourse once a week, if that often. Result? He developed severe prostatic symptoms —frequency of urination, pelvic pain, and, later on, complete impotence, because his overworked prostate gland finally could not keep up the pace.

Then there was the thirty-nine-year-old lawyer who claimed that he had had sex at least once a day (over the weekend it would be more often) for all of the fifteen years of his married life. He showed up now with a full-blown prostatitis, and when I suggested that as part of his treatment he would have to cut down on his sex activity, he refused, saying this was his "life style" and he "would rather die."

Quite a few of my patients have been young adolescents who, having learned the pleasure of masturbation, have repeated it daily or several times a day only to have a progressive buildup of prostatic changes.

I remember one seventeen-year-old high-school student who was shy with girls and indulged his sexual desires by daily masturbation. He became so frightened by urethral discharge and pain on voiding that he finally told his parents about his symptoms. When all three came to my office, the parents were astounded that prostate trouble could occur at seventeen; the boy himself could not believe his masturbation had caused his symptoms. Full explanations about his problem followed by a change in the boy's habit brought about improvement.

I also treat many young men, usually in their twenties, who stretch out the sexual act by holding their erections as long as possible before coming to a climax in ejaculation. Now sexual excitement involves blood filling not only of the penis but of all the pelvic organs, including the prostate. When the prostate is continually subjected to this swollen condition, it becomes inflamed.

So is it always from either too much or too little sex?

No, congestive prostatitis may develop without either abstinence or excessive sexual activity. A man in his late forties or in his fifties may develop it even though he has good sexual habits, apparently for no other reason than aging. It seems that among the many penalties of advancing years are various degenerative changes of the prostate.

How do you know you have congestive prostatitis?

Symptoms are many and varied:

Because the prostate is located at the bladder exit, a man may feel burning on urination and he may have to urinate more frequently than usual, even getting up from sleep to go to the toilet.

Other men may notice some discharge of a thin, whitish substance from the urethra.

Others may have pain in the lower back, groin, testicles, or thighs.

Some men discover something is wrong when they have sexual intercourse: a supersensitive inflamed prostate may trigger a premature ejaculation. Their semen may be streaked with blood or be quite bloody. Or they may have pain just after ejaculating.

Some men may be impotent to a greater or lesser degree—they will not be able to sustain an erection long enough to permit insertion into the vagina.

Is it always easy to tell when you have congestive prostatitis?

When prominent symptoms like those mentioned above are present, most men quickly realize that they have a problem, seek medical attention, and are quickly diagnosed. Yet some men with prostatic disorders do not have such obvious symptoms. As a result, they may not be aware that a urogenital problem exists and so do not seek medical help. This is especially true if a man has only a *slight* degree of impotence or trouble with ejaculation and feels too embarrassed about bringing it to his doctor's attention—often he waits until the symptoms become severe enough to cause him alarm.

In fact, even when a man does have a general checkup, his physician may overlook a urogenital disturbance. Not all general practitioners or internists are as alert to problems in this area as the urologist is.

How could a doctor overlook prostatitis?

Many a nagging, chronic, dull, low backache can be treated for years as an orthopedic or spine problem or as arthritis, neuritis, or sciatica. But there is no relief, until one day the prostate is examined and the cause is found there.

Similarly, persistent rectal discomforts—a feeling of fullness or of wanting to defecate often, or a rectal ache or pain—can make a man's life miserable until his prostatitis is found and treated.

All of this is true because the complex nerve supply of the pelvis and prostate may cause symptoms in the neighboring regions and organs although the primary problem lies in the prostate gland. A physician may therefore be easily confused about exactly where the trouble originates and may be diverted from making a correct diagnosis.

INFECTIOUS PROSTATITIS

How does the prostate become infected?

Inflammation of the prostate is very often due to bacterial attack. This is because the prostate is a gland of low resistance, particularly vulnerable to infection—a fact especially true if congestion of the prostate has been present beforehand. Such infections vary from low-grade chronic types to severe acute forms that can develop into abscesses.

In the past, gonorrheal infection was the most frequent cause of bacterial prostatitis. The germs spread from the original site in the urethra into the prostate, producing a fairly serious acute inflammation. But this type of infection is rare today. Although gonorrhea of course still exists, antibiotics usually control the infection in the urethra before it has a chance to spread to the prostate.

Occasionally gonorrhea proves resistant to antibiotics and is not completely overcome; then the germs do enter the prostate. However, in such a case the infection is now less severe than formerly. Sometimes it is so mild that the victim has no symptoms, nothing to warn him he is still diseased; the man then becomes a carrier of gonorrhea, infecting his sexual partner.

Germs in *any* part of the body may be transported by the blood to the prostate. Therefore infectious prostatitis often arises after respiratory ailments (bronchitis, flu, pneumonia, even a bad cold), sinus infections, or gastrointestinal ailments (such as diarrhea).

Bacteria may also spread from a kidney infection: infected urine coming from the bladder passes across the prostatic ducts, and extends right into the prostate. Kidney tuberculosis bacilli may be carried by the urine not only to the prostate but also to the other genital organs. Tuberculosis of the prostate rarely exists by itself—most often the seminal vesicles, the epididymis, and the testicles also become involved. Fortunately, we now have found many drugs effective against TB germs, so that urogenital tuberculosis can be controlled and cured.

Is it true you can catch prostatitis through sexual intercourse?

Apart from gonorrhea, there is another infection transmitted through intercourse that can cause prostatitis. Not infrequently a woman acquires a vaginal infection caused by a trichomonas organism; this is often a woman-to-woman infection, communicated through a contaminated toilet seat. The woman can pass on this rather troublesome one-celled invader to her male partner during sexual intercourse: the trichomonas organisms in the vagina enter the male urethra and travel up it to infect the prostate. (This organism cannot be transmitted by mouth.) Although this particular microscopic protozoan is very stubborn and resists treatment in both sexes, recent medication has made a cure reasonably certain. Both partners must be fully cured, for, if one is not, a Ping-Pong reaction may have them passing these organisms back and forth.

What are the symptoms of an acute prostatic infection?

Symptoms of infectious prostatitis vary quite a bit, depending on the cause and severity of the infection. An acute form may produce high fever, chills, frequent urination, burning, and pain on voiding. Pus and sometimes drops of blood may come from the penis at the end of urination. In any case, the symptoms of an acute attack are severe enough (and often painful enough) so that a man is quickly aware that he is ill.

Prompt treatment with antibiotics or other medication will take care of the high fever and general illness, but less prominent urinary symptoms may persist, indicating chronic prostatitis. Even if he has no further symptoms, a man who has had an acute phase of prostatitis should be checked later to be sure he has not developed a chronic, low-grade prostatitis.

How do you know you have a chronic infection?

With chronic infectious prostatitis, the symptoms—essentially the same as those of congestive prostatitis—are less dramatic. A man may have only urinary symptoms, such as urethral discharge or urinary frequency. Or he may have bladder symptoms *and* some sexual problem. Since a prostatic inflammation, like congestive prostatitis, may affect sites distant from the prostate, a man's symptoms may instead be those usually associated with neuritis and arthritis, confusing both patient and doctor. For this reason, a thorough physician treating an arthritic or neuralgic patient will try to uncover sources of infection in the teeth, tonsils, sinuses, or prostate.

How do abscesses form?

An abscess can develop from an acute (or even chronic) prostatitis, if the tiny infected areas break down and coalesce into a cavity that contains pus. Abscesses are rather rare today, because of the many antibiotics available to treat infections before they become this severe.

At times, just like a boil on the skin, the abscess may come to a head, break open of its own accord, and empty out through the urethra. This may occur whether antibiotics are given or not.

Rarely, an abscess will form and fail to rupture; in such cases, an operation is necessary.

I remember a diabetic patient who developed a high fever, severe burning, and frequency of urination. I not only found pus in his urine sample, but on rectal examination I discovered that his prostate was so full of pus that it was soft and bulging, and extremely tender. I felt that a barrelful of antibiotics would not help such a large abscess. This was one of the rare cases in which I had to operate for infection. Yet, after I got out almost a cupful of foul-smelling pus, the patient made a fine recovery. So even the most severe infections are amenable to treatment.

Does inflammation lead to prostatic stones?

Many men have stones along with prostatitis—one ailment propagates the other and aggravates the other's symptoms. Stones are also sometimes found along with enlargement of the prostate, and sometimes with prostatic cancer—or they may exist alone.

Stones are hard concretions, usually composed mainly of calcium, and are similar to many kidney or bladder stones. They may be as small as grains of sand or as large as cherry pits; generally multiple, they tend to cluster in nests. We don't know why they form in the prostate.

When a rectal examination reveals very hard nodules in the prostate, the physician probably will not know whether these nodules are stones or cancer or the two together. Only additional studies—which may include X ray, cystoscopy (a bladder examination), and occasionally biopsy of the prostate (removal and examination of a sample bit of tissue)—will yield a true diagnosis.

When stones exist alone and have not produced complaints, they need not be treated. If they are present along with chronic prostatitis, the symptoms may disappear if only the inflammation is treated. If this does not work, an operation to remove the stones must be done.

If stones exist along with enlargement of the prostate, the stones are removed as part of the operation for prostatic hypertrophy.

TREATMENT

What is the treatment for an inflamed prostate?

In treating either the infectious or congestive type of prostatic inflammation, our chief aims are to reduce the swelling (congestion) and to eliminate the accumulated inflammatory and breakdown products in the stored fluid.

The most vital part of treatment is prostatic massage —the physician inserts a finger into the rectum and presses against the prostate at several points to strip or squeeze it. The term "massage" is really a misnomer, for the doctor does not *rub* the gland—he presses a finger into it as you might press against a sponge to empty it. Massage empties the stored secretions from the gland. A congested gland feels doughy and boggy; but as the secretions drain out and improvement occurs, the prostate becomes normally firm. (If you touch the tip of your nose, you will know about how a healthy prostate feels.) Prostatic massage must be repeated at intervals;

following massage, microscopic examination of the fluid that is forced out will show what progress there has been in reducing the inflammation.

Antibiotics or other antibacterial medications are often given temporarily, especially when infection is present. Medication, however, is not a substitute for prostatic massage, for only by squeezing the gland can we get rid of the accumulated deteriorated fluid.

Is it true that you shouldn't drink?

Alcohol—whether whisky, wine, or beer—irritates the prostate, especially if a man drinks daily and in large amounts. Cutting down on drinking is therefore very important. Alcohol finds its way to all tissues of the body, including the prostatic fluid, where it aggravates any inflammation already present. In addition, alcohol in the urine irritates the lining of the prostatic urethra.

Spices and condiments have a similar though lesser effect, so such things as pepper, mustard, and hot sauces should be reduced or eliminated temporarily, too.

What about sex?

The frequency of sexual activity should be limited to once or twice a week, but total abstinence is not recommended. Some masturbation or intercourse—which are the same thing so far as the prostate is concerned—is good because ejaculation helps empty the prostate. Yet excess sexual activity only forces the already sick prostate to keep manufacturing fluid when it really needs a temporary rest period. What is more, sex should be in the form of a "quickie," for prolonged sexual excitement will engorge all of the sexual organs with blood and increase prostatic congestion.

What else can be done?

A man with prostatitis should also take hot baths frequently, sitting in the tub some ten to fifteen minutes each time. These baths give a great deal of comfort, especially if he has backache and lower abdominal discomfort.

Here are a few important don'ts:

Don't try a do-it-yourself prostatic massage. Rectal self-manipulation can cause severe damage to the delicate lining of the rectum. Leave this to your doctor, whether he is a general practitioner, internist, or urologist.

Don't be misled by patent medicines—either oral preparations or rectal suppositories. Not one has any beneficial effect; not one can cure prostatitis. Remedies advertised and virtually guaranteed to cure rectal, prostatic, urinary, or sexual problems are a complete waste of money. Diuretics or "kidney pills" and prostatic rectal suppositories benefit only the manufacturer and won't do you a bit of good. Fortunately, they contain little medication that has *any* effect on the body, so they won't poison you either; but if using them causes you to delay seeking proper medical diagnosis and treatment, you can aggravate your ailment.

Don't fall for devices for rectal irrigation or shortwave applications. These are of dubious, if any, value and could well make the inflammation worse.

Are operations ever done for prostatitis?

Don't be afraid that just because you have a prostate condition you will need an operation. Surgery is not necessary for simple prostatitis, and your doctor will tell you so—don't fear to consult him. As a matter of fact, even if acute prostatitis should completely shut off your urine, an operation is not necessarily called for. If urine blockage happens in the acute, high-fever type of prostatitis, we need only treat the infection. Similarly, even when severe bladder symptoms indicate that the prostate is blocking the urine, this does not mean that the gland is permanently enlarged. Often the swelling is temporary. In such cases massage and other non-surgical treatment will reduce the swelling; as the prostate decreases in size, the blockage of urine lessens, too.

In fact, surgical removal of the prostate for simple prostatitis would leave behind the inflamed tissue of the prostatic capsule, so that urinary or other symptoms would persist even after the operation. Surgery (except in rare cases) is not the answer for prostatitis.

3. Enlargement of the Prostate

A 3 A.M. telephone call:

"Doctor, you must do something! My husband can't pass his urine at all—he's in agony."

"How long has this been going on?"

"Well, all day yesterday he was passing only small amounts of urine, and after eight in the evening he couldn't pass any at all. He's in terrible pain."

"How old is he?"

"Seventy-seven."

"Has he had any prior trouble?"

"No, just the usual things at his age—getting up a few times at night and going a lot in the daytime—but that's expected, isn't it, when a man grows older?"

"Not exactly. However, you'll have to bring him to the hospital now, and we'll have to put a tube into his bladder to drain his urine."

This type of emergency is all too common in the work of urologists. The patient had benign enlargement of the prostate, the most frequent disorder of the prostate gland, and had ignored the early symptoms.

Benign enlargement, which tends to hit the older man, differs from inflammations of the prostate in that it is irreversible. In other words, while the swelling of congestive or infectious prostatitis occurs from within the prostate gland, it is usually a temporary condition alleviated by drugs, massage, and other nonsurgical means—benign enlargement is a *growth* of the lobes of the gland itself.

Isn't it normal to have trouble urinating as you get older?

This is a popular misconception. Age may make you gray or weak, but it does not cause you to get up at night to urinate. Only a disorder of your prostate makes you do that.

Mistaken notions that urinary frequency is normal in a man who has passed middle age make many men ignore early warning signs of impending prostatic trouble—particularly because such trouble is insidious; it creeps up on a man. Any symptom of urinary disorder should be brought to your doctor's attention. (See Chapter 5 for a list of guidelines.)

But isn't prostatic enlargement inevitable with aging?

Not at all. Prostatic enlargement does come in later years. About 10 percent of all fifty-year-old men have some growth of the prostatic lobes, and the ailment becomes more common as men age, affecting about half of all men seventy or older.

But this growth is *not* inevitable since only half of all men, even in their eighties, show any sign of it at all. So age is not the entire answer.

How does the prostate cause urinary problems?

We don't know why, but as *some* men age, a number of the prostatic glands located around the urethra begin to grow and form separate rounded masses, or lobes, which slowly progress in size. (Generally, two enlarging lobes appear, one on each side, but often a middle lobe develops as well.)

As these lobes enlarge they compress the urethra, slowly closing off the channel where it comes out of the bladder. As the urine can no longer flow freely, the bladder empties slowly or inefficiently, resulting in the symptoms described in Chapter 5.

What makes these lobes grow?

We don't really know, but one likely reason is an imbalance in hormone production. We know for certain that eunuchs, who have never been able to produce

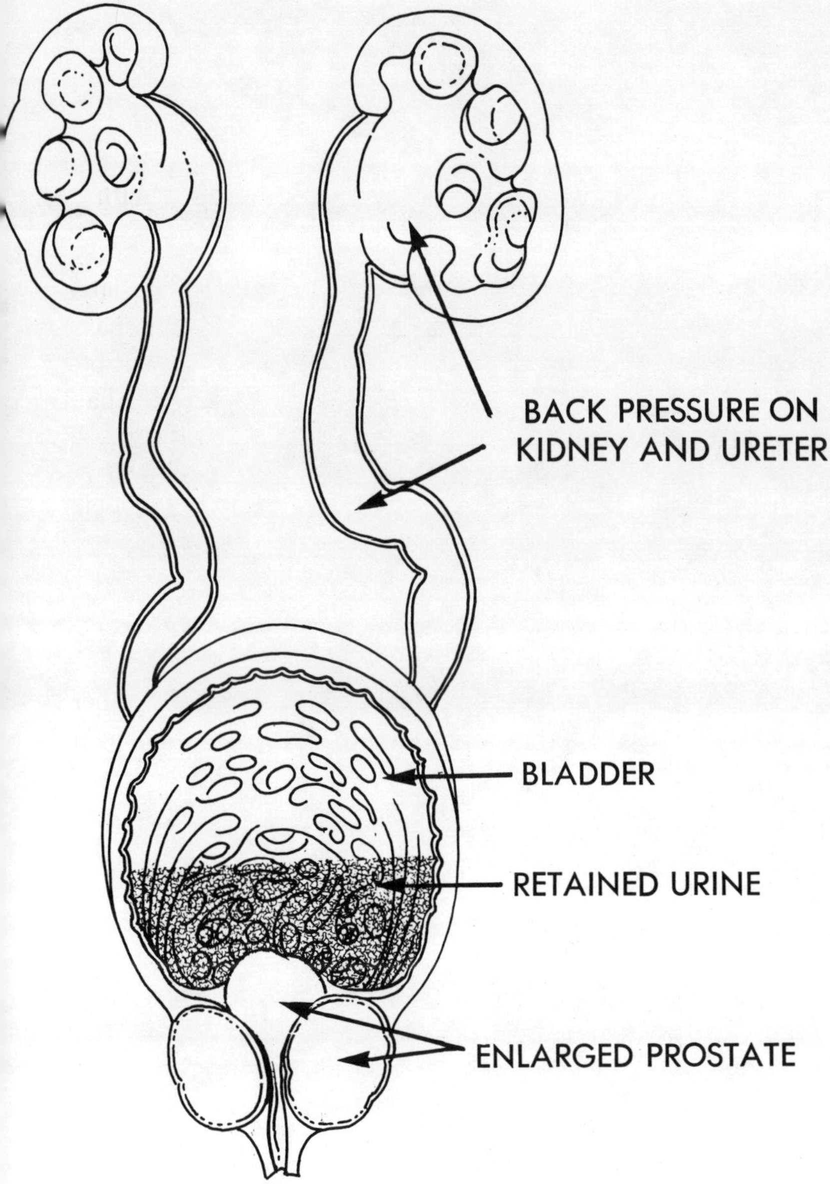

Enlargement of the prostate: When prostatic lobes enlarge, they compress the urethra, blocking the urine. The urine can back up the ureters to the kidneys, eventually ballooning them out and damaging them.

testosterone, never develop prostatic growth. Although this would lead one to assume that testosterone causes abnormal enlargement of the prostate, this is not wholly true either. Research studies show that patients with prostatic enlargement do *not* have excess testosterone. Also, if male hormones alone were responsible for prostatic enlargement, you would expect that administration of female sex hormones might reduce the growth. But female hormones don't seem to have any significant effect. The answer may lie in a delicate imbalance of various hormones, though the male and female sex hormones may play the major role.

Is prostatic enlargement a form of cancer?

Cancer and enlargement are quite different ailments. Cancer cells (as I explain more fully in Chapter 4) are not normal parts of the prostatic tissue; they are a wild, independent growth with the power to spread beyond the prostate to other parts of the body.

The growth of prostatic lobes, in contrast, involves normal prostatic tissue. Though the enlarged lobes cause trouble by physically pressing against the urethra, the growth remains within the prostatic capsule and cannot invade tissues elsewhere in the body.

Isn't an enlarged prostate caused by having masturbated as a boy?

No. This is a myth.

It is also untrue that prostatic enlargement is caused

by single or multiple attacks of gonorrhea or by sexual excesses. Indeed, even celibates, such as priests, develop it. Sexual practices have no bearing on the growth of this gland.

Can young men ever get this kind of urinary blockage?

While prostatic enlargement is generally a malady of older men, another type of growth that blocks the urine, called median bar, can afflict boys or men of any age. Median bar, though it differs from prostatic enlargement in origin and symptoms, can also lead to kidney damage and other consequences of obstruction.

What is median bar?

Median bar does not develop with advancing age but can be present at birth (in which case it is a developmental defect or abnormality). It is not rare in childhood or adolescence and is often found in young adult men.

Although it is similar in effect to enlargement of the middle lobe of the prostate, median bar is not a true enlargement of the prostate itself. It is actually a condensation of fibrous or scar tissue—in the shape of a bar—across the point where the urethra leaves the bladder. This scar tissue can form when an infection of the neck of the bladder heals. Just as a dam blocks water behind it, median bar obstructs the bladder exit, trapping urine in the bladder.

What are the symptoms of median bar?

Median-bar blockage is often insidious; even though it progressively blocks urinary outflow and backs the urine up to the kidneys, it seldom produces prominent symptoms. This is one of the faults of nature: it sometimes does not call attention to illness. You may have heard of "walking pneumonia"—an illness in which someone has pneumonia and is not aware of it—or of cases in which a person has a heart problem for some time without symptoms, and then has a sudden heart attack. The absence of symptoms in many ailments fails to alert the patient, and thus the problem cannot be detected early. Unfortunately, this is also true of median bar.

If there are no symptoms, how is it detected?

There are times when median bar does produce frequency of urination and having to get up at night just as prostatic enlargement does. This of course alerts the man. At other times, though no urinary symptoms are present, a physician finds a greatly distended bladder, like a blown-up balloon, across the lower abdomen. The bladder has slowly distended for months or even years as the median bar has permitted only part, not all, of the urine to pass at each voiding.

Isn't enlargement of the prostate a minor problem as long as the urine isn't blocked off completely?

Definitely not. Benign enlargement and median bar can cause kidney damage, which is fatal if not treated, and other serious problems. And an additional danger of ignoring urinary symptoms is that they can be signs not only of benign prostatic enlargement but also of cancer.

How does urinary blockage cause kidney damage?

As you probably know, the kidneys produce urine by filtering the blood to remove waste products, especially urea, which is formed when proteins (found in all meat, fish, eggs, and cheese, and some other foods) are broken down by the body. The urine flows down from the kidneys through the ureters to the bladder, where it is temporarily stored. The bladder, composed of crisscrossing layers of muscle, normally holds about a glassful of urine, but when stretched thin, it can accommodate up to about a quart. In a few extreme cases, a human bladder has been able to contain up to about a gallon.

When something happens to block the outflow of urine, the muscles of the bladder first become thickened and stronger in an attempt to expel the urine. But should the obstruction, such as from an increasingly enlarging prostate or median bar, continue, even the thickened, stronger bladder muscle is no longer able to eject all the urine. Some remains in the bladder after voiding. It then backs up, gradually reaching the kidneys, where it presses on and balloons out the functioning tissue, and by this backward pressure destroys it. If this process goes on long enough, the kidneys become badly damaged and lose their ability to filter the wastes from the blood properly. Then urea piles up in the blood. Since urea and other waste products are poisonous, this condition, known as uremia, is fatal if not treated. A delay in treating the growing, obstructing lobes of the prostate, or median bar, can lead to death.

It is therefore vital to remedy blockage in its early stages. Fortunately, as more men become aware that urinary problems are not a normal sign of aging but a danger signal, they are consulting their doctors at the earliest symptoms of prostatic obstruction. As a result more men today receive treatment before kidney destruction occurs.

What are the other dangers of an enlarged prostate?

Retained urine in the bladder can be compared to the water in a swamp, where drainage does not occur. Like any stagnant collection of water, which becomes dirty and foul with many putrid growths, retained urine becomes infected with bacteria. More than this, the infection may spread to the kidneys, creating an even more serious problem.

Also, when urine stagnates in the bladder, the crystals

that are ordinarily present may precipitate out and agglutinate together, forming stones. These may increase blockage to urinary outflow if they fall against the exit path from the bladder. Stones, moreover, invite infection, which in turn tends to create more stone formation. It is a never-ending vicious circle.

If the kidneys are damaged, one result may be the additional handicap of high blood pressure; back pressure of the blocked urine makes the injured kidney tissue produce a substance called renin, which raises blood pressure.

As if all of this were not enough, we find that patients with heart conditions are indirectly made worse because these men have the problems of straining to void and getting up at night.

What can be done for an enlarged prostate?

Almost all the effects of prostatic enlargement and median-bar obstruction are almost completely reversible if the blockage is removed before these effects become far advanced.

Though a better understanding of hormones may open up new treatments in the future, at present the only treatment for either enlargement or median bar is surgical. In such an operation, we usually do not remove the prostate itself, but only the obstructing lobes or the median bar. (Chapter 8, "Operations of the Prostate," details the several techniques.)

In some cases, we can't operate right away. If kidney damage is severe, for instance, the bladder may first have to be drained by a tube, or catheter, for a varying time. Also, we may have to overcome infection before we can deal with the prostatic problem itself.

Once the obstruction has been removed, however, and the stagnant urine released, infection tends to recede. Stones are of course removed during the same operation. Most important of all, removal of the blockage means there is no longer any backing up of the urine. The kidneys, free of back pressure, are again able to remove urea and other waste products from the blood. If no damage has been done to the kidneys, they continue functioning as they have always done.

What if the kidneys have already been damaged?

The kidneys show a most surprising capacity to heal themselves. I have operated on many patients with greatly damaged kidneys to find that after several months their kidneys had completely recovered the ability to cleanse their blood of waste products.

4. Cancer of the Prostate

Stanley was terrified when I told him he had cancer of the prostate. He'd always been so healthy he hadn't been to a doctor in twenty years. Now, in his early sixties, he had come to me only because he was having a little trouble urinating.

"That's impossible," he said, when I explained that his cancer was so extensive it was too late to cure. "I haven't had any symptoms until now."

"It's a silent disease," I said. "Often there are no symptoms in the early stages." I explained that a total cure was impossible because it was too late to remove the prostatic cancer—the malignant growth had spread beyond the prostate. X rays clearly showed it was already in the bones.

Stanley, like many patients who hear they have cancer, immediately assumed he would soon die.

> "Not for a good long while," I assured him. "I can promise you years of comfortable life—you could die of any number of other things before this cancer. It's a paradox—medicine cannot cure you, yet you can have years to live."

How frequent is cancer of the prostate?

Almost twenty thousand Americans will probably die of prostatic cancer each year during the 1970's. This cancer is not common in young men, but it is the third leading cause of death due to cancer in men over the age of fifty-five; only cancer of the lung and of the lower intestine are more frequent. After the age of seventy-five, prostatic cancer becomes the leading cause of death from malignant disease. Cancer, in fact, is the third most frequent ailment of the prostate after inflammation and benign enlargement.

What causes cancer of the prostate?

Cancer is a type of cell that disregards all rules of normal growth; such cells multiply prolifically, forming lumps (tumors). But perhaps even more important, cancer cells have the power to invade surrounding tissues and organs, breaking through the usual barriers such as tissue capsules or envelopes. They are also capable of entering blood and lymph vessels, and can be swept by the blood or lymph streams to distant parts of the body. This spread or invasion is known as metastasis.

Just why normal cells go wild suddenly and form

a cancer is as yet unknown. We don't even know whether cancer results from a single cause, such as a virus, or has several complex causes. And this is true for cancer of the prostate as for other types of cancer.

Is it true that VD or too much sex can cause prostatic cancer?

Although we don't know the cause of prostatic cancer, we do know enough to demolish old wives' tales such as these. It is certainly *not* true that prostatic cancer is related to or caused by venereal disease, sexual excesses, abstinence, or masturbation. And although cancer can coexist with inflammation, stones, or enlargements, such problems are not forerunners of cancer. Many men who develop prostatic cancer have never had any prostatic difficulties in the past, and many men who *have* suffered other prostatic problems never develop cancer.

What are the symptoms?

In its early stages, prostatic cancer is "silent"—that is, it does not produce any complaints to warn a man of its presence. Because it generally starts at the outer edge of the gland, at a distance from the urethra, a man is not likely to have any early bladder signals such as frequent urination or bloody urine. As a result, a man may have cancer of the prostate for a long time before becoming aware of it or before his physician makes a rectal examination as a routine check.

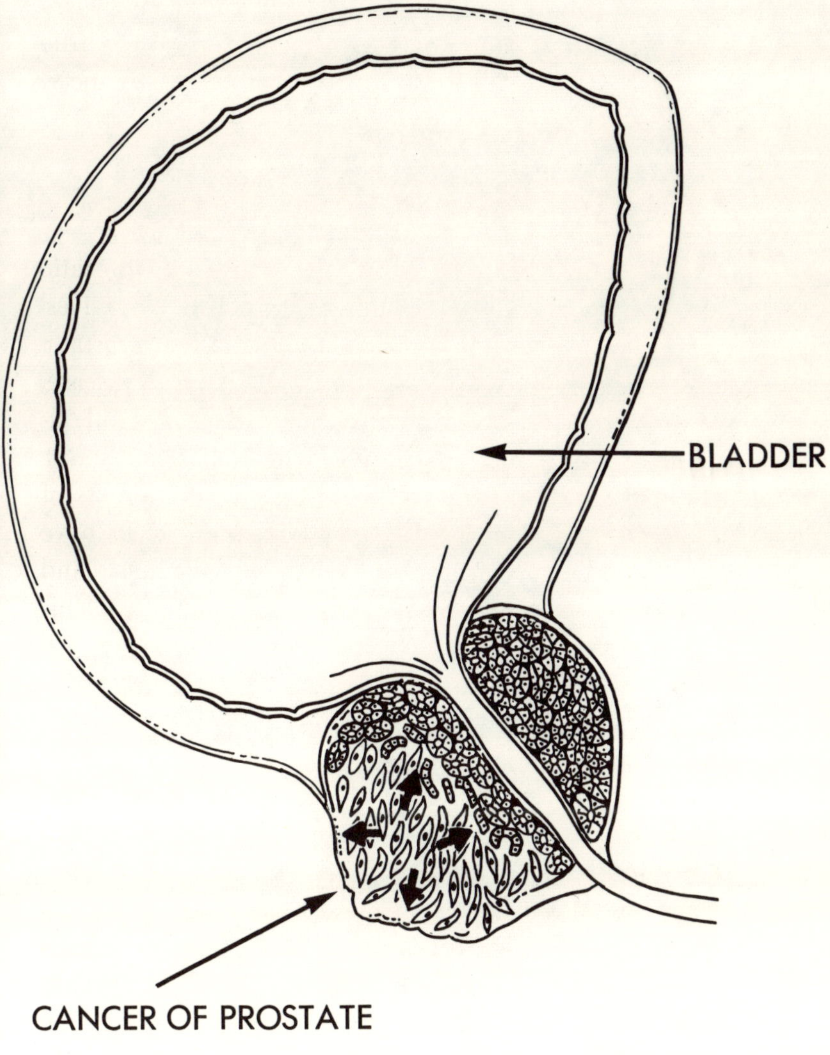

Cancer of the prostate: Cancer generally starts at the outer edge of the prostate gland, at a distance from the urethra.

Then how is it detected?

Since cancer of the prostate usually starts at the outer edge of the gland, just underneath the rectal wall, in most cases a physician can feel even an early tumor with his finger during a rectal examination. It feels like a hard nodule—a stone-hard, pea-sized bump on an otherwise smooth-surfaced gland. The diagnosis is confirmed by looking at some of the cells under the microscope. Cells for this purpose can be secured by biopsy—removal of a sample of tissue.

Regrettably few men have this examination on a regular basis, so early diagnosis is not frequent. This is unfortunate, since diagnosis before the cancer has spread offers the greatest chance for successful treatment and cure. Early cancer detection is a most important reason why men should have a rectal examination as a customary part of an annual checkup, especially from the age of fifty on.

How is a biopsy done?

Unfortunately, we cannot use such a simple technique as a Pap smear, which detects cancer of the uterus in women. Cells can be obtained for the Pap test through a woman's vagina by simply inserting a cotton-tipped applicator or a tiny rubber suction device.

To obtain a sample of tissue from the prostate, a physician has to insert a needle through the perineum (the area between the scrotum and anus) or rectum to the suspicious portion of the prostate gland. This requires at least a local anesthetic and at times may be unsuccessful because the tip of the needle may miss the exact spot needed. In some cases, a biopsy is made during surgery through the same perineal area.

How fast does it grow?

Cancer of the prostate is relatively slow-growing. It may even lie dormant for long periods. Exactly why it may suddenly burst into activity is not known. Because it advances slowly and because of excellent treatments available today, if a man *had* to choose one kind of cancer of those occurring frequently, cancer of the prostate would be the sanest choice. Nevertheless, no matter how slowly, ultimately the cancer does grow.

What happens when it spreads?

It may spread throughout the entire prostate gland. In doing so, it compresses the urethra and causes urinary-blockage symptoms similar to those of benign prostatic enlargement; even though a physician may suspect one or the other, he usually cannot make an absolute diagnosis without a biopsy.

A second effect is metastasis—the cancer may grow beyond the limit of the prostatic capsule and invade surrounding tissues. If it spreads underneath the bladder, it may choke the ureters (the tubes leading down from the kidneys). Urine will then back up to the kidneys, and the man will be in danger of uremia and uremic poisoning.

If, instead of invading the closest surrounding tissues, the cancer metastasizes to the lymph system, it can be carried to quite distant points. In fact, prostatic cancer cells have a predilection for entering the lymph vessels which ordinarily travel with nerves. As nerves are of course sensitive, a man can have considerable pain when lymph spread occurs. But the cancer does not necessarily stop here. Lymphatic vessels often carry the cancer to bones, for example, where they produce satellites or cancer metastases. Bones that seem especially vulnerable to attack by prostatic cancer are those of the lower spine and hip areas.

How does the lymphatic system disseminate cancer?

We understand much less about the lymphatic system than we do about the blood circulation system. The lymph system, consisting of ducts and glands, is generously distributed throughout the body; its tiny vessels transport a whitish fluid containing various substances important for bodily function. For example, the lymph vessels of the gastrointestinal tract carry many absorbed food elements.

The lymph channels are mostly delicate and very small, invisible to the naked eye; at intervals, there are way stations called lymph glands. These are barriers to invaders which are trying to advance throughout the body. They act as filters to stop bacteria, and they will even attempt to destroy cancer cells.

Very often, however, the lymph glands are unable to destroy the cancer cells. Instead, they themselves become enlarged with the cancerous growth, which then proceeds farther along the lymph channels, spreading itself through the body. In this way, cancer ultimately enters the blood stream through a large duct high in the chest just below the neck. From the blood stream, the cancer can of course be carried to every part of the body.

The lymphatic system also defends the body by producing some of the white blood cells and some antibodies. Antibodies are specialized substances, each one manufactured against a particular invader, such as specific bacteria, viruses, or even cancer cells. Our bodies begin to produce these antibodies after we have contracted an infectious disease, such as smallpox, polio, or flu, and will often continue producing antibodies so that we remain immune to the disease for a long time (in some cases, apparently, for the rest of our lives).

With smallpox and several other diseases, we are able to stimulate the production of the proper antibodies artificially, through inoculation, and thus avoid the disease altogether. Whether or not a cancer-fighting antibody can be isolated—and therefore an inoculation against cancer developed—is a question now being investigated by cancer research teams. But for the time being, we have no such simple solution.

How is cancer of the prostate treated?

The three basic treatments are surgery, radiation, and hormone therapy, but most men with prostatic cancer are treated with more than one of these methods.

Can surgery cure prostatic cancer?

If a man is lucky enough, his annual physical examination will include a rectal examination, and cancer of the prostate would be diagnosed early: a biopsy would be done on the small hard nodule that feels like cancer and the diagnosis would be confirmed before the tumor had an opportunity to spread. The growth would be confined to the prostate and could be removed by radical prostatectomy, which includes the removal not only of the tumor, but of the entire prostate, its capsule, and the seminal vesicles (see Chapter 8).

Unfortunately, although this operation can result in a complete cure, few patients benefit from this treatment because most men do not get to their doctors early enough. In most cases, by the time a man gets into treatment the cancer has already extended into the tissues outside the prostatic capsule.

Occasionally, even if the prostatic cancer has already spread, we can give hormonal treatment, which shrinks the growth down to manageable form; then it is sometimes possible to perform radical prostatectomy. Regrettably, we cannot do this very often—only in about 5 percent of cancer cases is it possible to reduce the cancer to a small enough size. My own opinion is that radical prostatectomy should be reserved for the younger man whose cancer is in an early stage. The elderly man can be successfully treated with alternate methods.

Does this surgery have any special risks?

One risk of radical prostatectomy is that it sometimes damages the urinary control muscles—the urethral sphincters—so that the man becomes incontinent. However, this is a small risk to take in exchange for the total removal of cancer. A more upsetting disadvantage is that most men become impotent following this kind of operation (see Chapter 10 for further information about impotence).

What can be done if it's too late for surgery?

Once prostatic cancer has spread so that surgery cannot remove all of it, we can use other forms of treatment, or sometimes surgery *plus* other treatments. For instance, we can first remove the blocking portion of the cancer to eliminate retention of urine. This need not involve an abdominal incision but can be done by the ingenious transurethral method (described in Chapter 8), in which instruments are inserted through the penis to the prostatic area; electrical currents cut away tissue and coagulate or cauterize any blood vessels that are met in the cutting process. After this type of surgery a man is generally given some other form of treatment as well, such as hormone therapy.

What is hormone therapy?

In the 1890's, some men with enlarged prostates were treated by removal of both testicles; some improved, some did not, but nobody knew why. It was not until

1941 that the brilliant American investigator Dr. Charles Huggins, who later won a Nobel Prize for his research, wondered whether this approach might work for men with prostatic cancer.

Among Dr. Huggins' discoveries was that cancerous prostatic tissues contain fairly large amounts of a certain enzyme, acid phosphatase. Since acid phosphatase is not found at all in the prostates of eunuchs or preadolescent boys, but is found in small amounts in normal adult men, Dr. Huggins reasoned that the production of this enzyme is connected with sexual maturity. As the levels of acid phosphatase are highest of all in prostatic cancer, he thought that growth of prostatic cancer might be dependent upon a supply of male sex hormone. By cutting off the supply of this hormone, therefore, he thought he might be able to reduce prostatic cancer growth. This proved true: when men with advanced cancer had their testicles removed, they greatly improved and were dramatically relieved of pain.

A similar relationship seems to exist in women, as the removal of the ovaries (the organs producing female sex hormones) has been found helpful in many cases of breast cancer.

This concept that certain cancers are dependent on sex hormones for their wild growth provided what is now one of the major methods of attack on prostatic cancer. Even when cancer has metastasized to the bones, it is possible to slow down its growth by removing male sex hormone. A reversion toward normal occurs not only in the prostate but in the invaded area as well—no matter how far from the prostate.

A side effect of these discoveries was the realization

that it is generally most unwise for a physician to prescribe male sex hormone to any man complaining of poor sexual ability; extra testosterone may light up an area of latent cancer in the prostate and stimulate it to active growth.

Is castration the only means of eliminating hormone activity?

It is also possible to counteract the effect of male sex hormone by giving pills or injections of female sex hormones. For some patients this will be done in addition to removing the testicles, but in other cases only female sex hormone will be given.

What about the male sex hormones produced elsewhere in the body?

Although the testicles produce most of a man's testosterone, similar male sex hormones are supplied by other organs, particularly the adrenal glands. In some men, therefore, not only are the testicles surgically removed, but also the adrenals; in a very few cases, the pituitary (a gland at the base of the brain) is surgically destroyed, too.

For about 80 percent of men with prostatic cancer, however, castration and the use of female sex hormones will be enough to keep the cancer under control.

Will hormone therapy cure cancer?

Yes and no. We are never certain that all of the cancer cells have been suppressed or killed. On the other hand, many men continue to live with this treatment until they eventually die of other ailments and are thus seemingly cured of cancer.

Will hormone therapy put an end to sex?

Not necessarily. An adult man doesn't need to have testicles to have intercourse; even without them he can continue to have erections. Taking estrogens also will not necessarily rule out sex. Undoubtedly, castration or estrogen therapy will *reduce* sexual activity in most men, but as the mechanism for erection and sexual ability remains intact, many men continue to be sexually active. The least impairment of sexual capacity is in those men who receive female sex hormone only and who retain their testicles.

Do female hormones have any side effects?

Chances are that a man's breasts will enlarge slightly and his nipples will get a little tender. Most men tolerate this as a minor inconvenience (which it is). But if a man thinks he would be bothered by this slight enlargement, he can avoid it by a small dose of X-ray treatment before starting the estrogens. In the rare case in which a man would find enlarged breasts unusually upsetting, or feel himself disfigured, we can remove some of the breast tissue surgically.

Is there any way a man can hide the fact that his testicles are missing?

Silicone plastic implants can be inserted on each side at the time the testicles are removed. These harmless, inert implants give the effect of normal testicles; they can therefore be very beneficial to a man who feels he is disfigured and who would be very self-conscious in a gym locker room or at a beach, for example. The replacement plastic testicle is available everywhere and is not as uncommon as you might think. It is made of the same material used by cosmetic surgeons to increase the size of women's breasts.

Are there other treatments besides surgery and hormone therapy?

Recently, supervoltage radiation therapy—generally, cobalt radiation—has given us another method to attack cancer. This is the same type of X ray used routinely (for chest X rays, for example), except that it is enormously more powerful. Ordinary X rays have a "jolt" or energy of up to 150,000 electron volts; the beams for cancer treatment, derived from other sources (especially nuclear energy, such as from radioactive cobalt), have an impact up to many million electron volts. The radiation beams are finely aimed at the deep prostatic-cancer areas; they have an advantage over the lower-potency X-ray beams because they cause less damage to the skin and other tissues surrounding the prostate.

Although it is particularly suited to cancer that is still fairly limited, radiation can also be directed at any bone to which the cancer has spread. Thus a cancer-killing dose of radiation can be given to either early or far-advanced cancer patients.

Can drugs be used on prostatic cancer?

Drugs have been developed to counteract various types of malignant growth: leukemia and Wilms' tumor of the kidney have been successfully treated in this way. Unfortunately, despite much research, no drug (except female sex hormone) has yet been developed for prostatic cancer.

What about the future?

Needless to say, researchers continue to try new approaches. As one example, still on an experimental basis, radioactive gold is injected into the prostatic cancer at open surgery in doses large enough to kill cancer cells. The gold continues to emit radioactive rays for months and so has a continuing action against the cancerous growth. This method is being tested at only a few medical institutions in this country, and we must have experience with many patients over a number of years before we can judge its effectiveness.

Radioactive drugs are also being used in cases in which castration and female sex hormones fail to halt cancer growth or do so only temporarily. Such men may experience a great deal of pain once prostatic cancer has spread to the bones. Here we can administer testosterone (*male* sex hormone) to stir up or further activate the painful bony cancer cells, then inject radioactive phosphorus into the blood stream. The blood deposits this radioactive phosphorus in the bones, where it emits rays destructive to the cancer cells.

This powerful radiation delivered directly to the pain-producing sites has been quite helpful to many patients.

Which treatment is the most effective?

Exactly what treatment a man will get depends on a variety of factors. A treatment that is effective in an early stage may not be so later, so a physician's choice has to depend on the nature of each patient's cancer. Just as men are individuals, so are their diseases—what works on one man's cancer may not work on another's, and usually a combination of treatments is tried until a special plan is evolved for each patient.

Far from being a hopeless case, a man with cancer of the prostate has many treatment possibilities. If surgery will not work, other methods can be used. We are still in an era when no one definitive therapy is available, but where several treatment efforts, each supplementing the other, can produce good results and keep a patient alive and comfortable for very long periods, generally for years.

5. Danger Signs of Prostatic Enlargement

"I guess I'm getting old," Kenneth told his doctor. "I have to go to the toilet all the time—even at night."

"That's an old wives' tale," said the doctor. "Urinary problems aren't normal no matter *how* old you are. That's your prostate kicking up."

As I explained in Chapter 3, urinary problems are not a normal sign of aging but danger signals of prostate disorders. A man developing an enlarged prostate might have any of the following symptoms:

Feeble urination

In general, when a man has prostate trouble, his urinary stream becomes feeble. When he's asked, "Can you urinate with as great force as when you were a youngster?" he answers, "No, it comes out slowly."

Frequent urination

Frequency of urination is easy to overlook for a while. A man developing prostatic problems will often unconsciously gear his habits to his new need to urinate frequently. When he goes driving, he plans to stop at a service station not only to buy gas but to go to the men's room. He automatically checks to see where the lavatory is when he first enters a restaurant. He is sure to go to the toilet before the picture begins at a cinema so that he will not have to get up during the show. At the theater, the intermission is a blessing to him—he can visit the men's room.

Slow or incomplete urination

Another symptom is that he can't start to urinate promptly—he has to stand and wait a bit—and when he finishes, some drops remain behind so that he has some final dribbling. Even then, he may not be sure he has emptied his bladder, and soon he may want to return to the toilet. He may at times be plagued by the urgent need to pass urine and then find it hard to void when the chance does come.

Getting up at night

This is also common and disturbing. First it's once a night. Later, even though a man may purposely try to cut down on fluids before retiring, he'll find he has to get up two or three times.

Passing blood

A more alarming symptom is passing blood with the urine. This happens because enlargement of the prostate swells the associated blood vessels. The stretched walls of these blood vessels may rupture, especially when the man has to strain to pass urine.

In most cases bleeding is minor—only a few drops of blood may show up the first time—then it may disappear, only to show up at a later time. However, the amount of bleeding varies. It may even reach the level of a full-blown hemorrhage and become a true emergency requiring immediate hospitalization to staunch the flow.

Inability to urinate

The urine may totally shut off most unexpectedly—and this also develops into a true emergency. This complete urinary retention is likely to occur after taking a few extra alcoholic drinks or with exposure to cold weather (for example, watching a football game or engaging in outdoor activity in winter).

Tiredness and nausea

When kidney damage has crept up all unknown, the man may have poor appetite and nausea, may feel dragged out and tired all the time. When and if our poor patient reaches this phase, he is sick indeed and most likely has ignored the much earlier warning symptoms of difficulties with urination.

I might add that all the symptoms described above can occur with prostatic blockage due either to cancerous or noncancerous growth of the prostate. Sometimes pain, especially in the low back, accompanies prostatic cancer, but symptoms alone will not distinguish between the two conditions. Only medical examination and study will diagnose whether the growth is malignant or benign.

6. Especially for Women—the Female Prostate

"Doctor, I remember when my father was in his late sixties, he had great difficulty passing his urine. Before he was operated on for his prostate he had to get up many times at night, and during the day he would go to the bathroom almost every hour. I have many bladder symptoms that resemble his. It can't be that I have prostate trouble, can it? Women don't have prostates, do they?"

What is the female prostate?

Many people are surprised to learn that women have a prostate. But every fetus—whether it is male or female—has a group of glands surrounding the upper portion of the urethra (the tube that leads away from the bladder). In men, these tiny glands enlarge until they develop into the prostate. In women, this tissue usually remains small, but it can sometimes grow enough to form an obstruction in the same place—at the neck (the exit) of the bladder. Thus a similar situation exists in both sexes.

Can a woman develop prostate problems?

A woman certainly may develop urinary symptoms as pronounced and prominent as any man's. Should the tissue at the neck of the bladder grow, it can block her outflow of urine to varying degrees. She may even have complete retention of urine so that she cannot void at all. So a woman, too, may have to have the blocking tissue surgically removed. Obviously, this happens less frequently in women than in men, but it is not unknown, not even rare in the experience of any active urologist. (It is most frequent in diabetic patients.)

Can a woman develop cancer of the prostate?

Luckily not. The analogous growth of obstructing tissue in women involves only those glands which in the man undergo benign (noncancerous) growth of the prostate.

How common is a female prostate?

Women's bladder symptoms usually are *not* caused by "prostate" or the formation of obstructing tissue.

Most cases of urinary frequency in women are due to other conditions, such as "dropped bladder" (properly called cystocele), narrowing of the urethra, or inflammation of the bladder (cystitis) or of the urethra (urethritis). Most of these urinary outlet problems are minor, can be effectively treated with antibiotics or other simple means, and do not require surgery.

7. You and Your Urologist

Bill, aged sixty-four, had been in good health most of his life, but a need to urinate frequently had crept up on him over the past year.

His friends told him not to worry—everyone, they said, got bladder troubles as he got older. But Bill's wife insisted he call the family physician.

"Nonsense," said the doctor. "Urinary complaints aren't normal at *any* age. They're warning signals. When can you come in?"

When should you see a urologist?

When you are not urinating properly—when you are urinating too slowly or too frequently or have some other complaint—it is time to see a doctor. You may choose to go to your internist or general practitioner, who may then refer you to a urologist, or you may go directly to a urologist.

You may also telephone the County Medical Society in your area and ask them to give you the name of a specialist in urology, or you may ask your local hospital to recommend a urologist.

What happens then?

Let's suppose that Bill has arrived at my office a bit anxious. Although urinary trouble has brought Bill to me, I first want to know his entire medical history.

Why is a medical history important?

I need to know about Bill's previous ailments and any operations, even those in childhood, because these might have a bearing on his present condition.

Also, since I may have to give him medication or even operate on him, I need to know whether he has any allergies, high blood pressure, diabetes, or other problems which might complicate or even rule out particular treatments.

Finally, I have to ask Bill some questions he may consider highly personal—about his sex life, his smoking, or his drinking. If Bill feels his sex life is unsatisfactory or that he drinks too much, he may be tempted to hedge his answers a bit, embarrassed to admit the truth even though he knows such matters affect his body.

But this is only part of the reason I take a history

first. I know that Bill, even if he appears intelligent or cocky, is apprehensive—of me or of what might be wrong with him. He may even have greatly exaggerated fears. So the history not only gives me information, it provides an opportunity for Bill and me to get to know each other.

Why is communication so vital?

It gives Bill a chance to size me up and, I hope, develop confidence in my concern and ability to help him.

For me it is equally important, if I am not to be misled, to learn how to interpret Bill's words. Of ten patients who tell me about a similar symptom or pain, three may exaggerate it out of all proportion, three may minimize it by pretending it is nothing—and only by understanding the personalities of my patients can I properly evaluate the real importance of their complaints.

How is a diagnosis made?

Once Bill and I have gotten through the above preliminaries, we are ready to discuss his current problem, and my questions now are an attempt to narrow the several possibilities to a diagnosis. Does Bill have burning on urination? Has he seen any blood in his urine? Is his urinary stream forceful or weak? Does he have to wait for a while before he can start urinating? Does he feel that he is able to empty his bladder when he passes urine?

Actually, there is almost a pattern in Bill's replies, so I am not surprised when he tells me that urination has modified his daily living so that toilet facilities have become of paramount concern wherever he goes. I am now ready to examine Bill physically.

What does the physical examination consist of?

Bill's internist has given him a general examination—he has checked his heart and lungs, eyes, ears, nose, mouth, and blood pressure. But I will pay more attention to the abdomen: Can I feel Bill's kidneys with my fingers after I have told him to breathe in and out? Does he have abdominal masses? Is his bladder so full that it can be felt through the abdominal wall? Are his external genitalia normal?

Next, I examine Bill's prostate by having him bend over so that I can insert my gloved finger easily into the rectum. This painless and most important feature of Bill's examination tells me how large his prostate is. Is it hard or soft? Is it bumpy? Is it rigid and fixed in position, or is it slightly movable? Is the rectal wall loosely or firmly attached to the prostate? Is the prostate symmetrical or is one lobe different from the other?

Why is a rectal examination insufficient?

Usually rectal examination is very revealing, but it may also occasionally be misleading.

Most of the time, when the prostate blocks the urine, the enlargement is toward the back (toward the rectum), and I can feel it with my finger. But if the enlargement is toward the front (into the bladder), I cannot feel that enlargement. Bill's prostate might also feel deceptively normal if his blockage results from a median bar—which, again, would be on the opposite side of the prostate from where my finger is. The same may be true of prostatic stones—they can be hidden deep where they cannot be felt.

A final pitfall in diagnosing solely with a rectal examination is cancer. Usually cancer areas are hard and located at the back of the prostate, where I can easily feel them with my finger. But sometimes cancer cells are *not* hard, and it is then impossible to feel them. I also would miss the cancer if, instead of being close to the surface as it usually is, it is deep in the prostate.

For all of these exceptions a rectal examination will not be enough, and Bill will have to have X ray or other diagnostic tests as well.

What other tests are likely to be part of the first examination?

Sometimes I have to examine the prostatic fluid under a miscroscope. To obtain a sample, I exert gentle pressure on the prostate to squeeze some of the fluid out onto a glass slide for a microscope preparation or into a test tube for laboratory growth (culture) of bacteria.

I also do a urinalysis on Bill, as I do on every patient.

Why is urinalysis important?

The urine contains all the products which are filtered from the blood by the kidneys. Urine is examined for

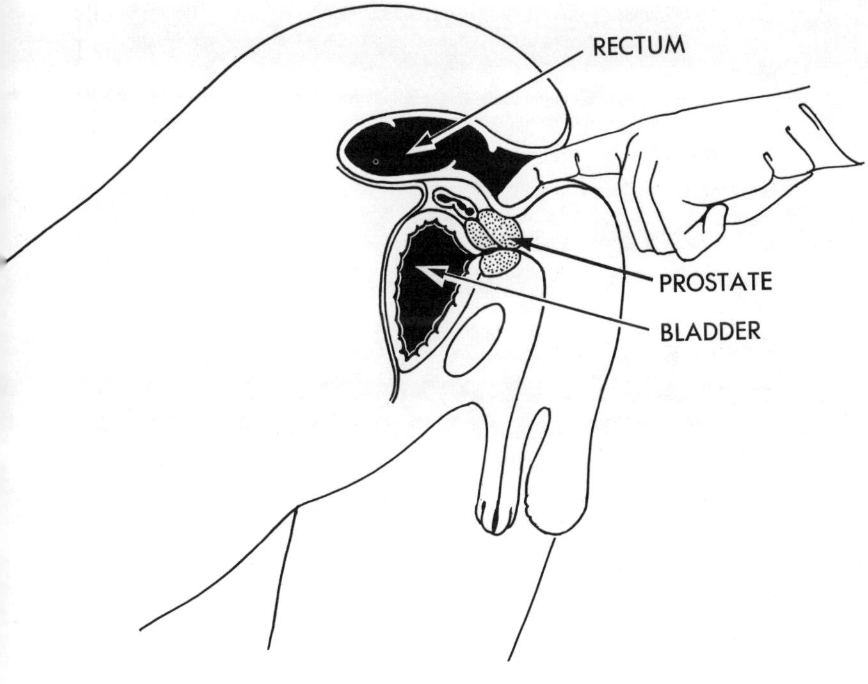

Examination of the prostate: Because the prostate is situated between the rectum and the bladder, a doctor can feel many types of abnormalities during a rectal examination.

abnormal components—albumin or sugar, pus cells, red blood cells, or other tiny structures shed by diseased kidneys.

Albumin or sugar in the urine indicates a general disease or an ailment of the kidneys themselves.

Pus cells in the urine show only that there is an inflammation or infection *somewhere* in the urinary tracts. Finding them does not pinpoint their origin—which might be the kidneys, ureters, bladder, prostate, or urethra—and further tests are necessary to find their source.

The same need for further tests is indicated by the presence of red blood cells which may be found under the microscope even when no blood can be seen in the urine with the naked eye.

To identify bacteria, urine is placed into a culture tube containing growth material for the germs. Tests can also be made to see which antibiotics or chemicals would best combat these bacteria.

Are there any other tests which are done as a matter of course?

At this time, having taken Bill's history, examined him, and done a urinalysis, I have a good idea of the diagnosis and I can also prescribe treatment. For example, I can be pretty sure whether Bill has prostatitis, enlargement of the prostate, or advanced cancer of the prostate. However, if what I have found up to this point is not enough for a diagnosis, or if I suspect some additional complications, there are other tests I might do. These include kidney function tests, blood studies, X rays, cystoscopy, and biopsies.

What are kidney function tests?

When I think that Bill's kidneys are not functioning well, there are a number of tests I might use to tell me exactly how well they *are* working. Since normal kidneys remove waste products from the blood, I can take samples of blood and urine from Bill. Comparing how much waste material the kidneys have transferred from the blood to the urine will give me the percentage of his kidney efficiency.

More extensive and sophisticated kidney tests can be done by injecting one of several chemicals, including some radioactive material, into a vein. I can then measure how much of these substances his kidneys have picked up and excreted. Such tests can tell me not only the type of kidney damage and its severity, but also, if repeated over a period of time, how his kidney disease is progressing.

What blood studies are done?

A blood count is important for detecting anemia; poor kidney function can be the basis for this thin blood. Moreover, if Bill is to have an operation, I will need to know whether he will require a transfusion beforehand, and his red blood count will help me determine how his general condition is.

A white blood count often shows the presence of infection somewhere in the body, since the white blood corpuscles are produced in great numbers when the body is trying to fight off bacteria.

There are many other blood tests that are not done routinely, but only for special reasons. If I contemplated operating on Bill, I might want to know whether his blood will clot normally or whether I would have to watch out for a bleeding tendency. Should I suspect Bill has cancer of the prostate, I would order a particular blood test. Very often, when cancer of the prostate has spread to the bones, the acid phosphatase level in the blood is higher than normal. When the cancer is confined to the gland, this blood acid phosphatase is normal. The test thus helps me determine whether metastasis has occurred.

When are X rays used?

Quite possibly, after completing Bill's physical examination plus urine or blood tests, I could be sure a blockage existed, and I would want X rays to show me the condition of his kidneys and bladder. These would also give me an excellent idea of how much the prostate is blocking the bladder outlet.

The intravenous pyelogram, or IVP, is perhaps the most valuable of all multiple types of X rays. I would inject a special iodine fluid into a vein in Bill's arm; this fluid would be collected by the kidneys from the blood, and, since this iodine medication makes a dense shadow on an X ray, it would outline his entire urinary tract from kidneys on down. This X-ray series gives us an idea of kidney function, informs us about blockage, shows us stones in either the kidneys or bladder, and even shows enlargement of the prostate when it pushes into the bladder. If I take an X ray right after Bill has urinated, I can see whether he has emptied his bladder completely or whether an obstruction, as from an enlarged prostate, is blocking the urinary flow.

What is cystoscopy?

Cystoscopy is another technique I might use on Bill if I wanted to take a look at his bladder and prostate without resorting to surgery. The cystoscope is basically a hollow tube which is inserted from the tip of the penis along the urethra into the bladder; the tube is wide enough to contain lenses and lighting apparatus. It's like a periscope—by looking at one end of the tube I can see whether Bill has a bladder tumor or a stone and how large his prostate is. If necessary, I could pass fine tubes called ureteral catheters up to the kidneys themselves for special testing. Should an operation on the prostate be necessary, cystoscopy can help me determine which type of operation would be best suited for Bill.

Is cystoscopy painful?

At one time it was, but no longer, and people should not fear this procedure. With today's local anesthetics and improved instruments, the cystoscopic examination is only a minor discomfort—so minor that it is performed frequently everywhere as a routine office test.

What is a biopsy?

This test involves the removal of tissue for microscopic examination and is performed only when we suspect cancer. A sample so small that it can be removed with a needle is large enough for the pathologist to determine whether the tissue is malignant.

Needle biopsy of the prostate can be done under local anesthesia and takes only a few minutes. It can be done in an office, but, like many other urologists, I prefer to do it in a hospital where the patient can be adequately medicated and where the biopsy is part of a full diagnostic study.

Is needle biopsy of the prostate foolproof?

Frankly, no. It is possible to miss the area or nodule you want; the needle tip may go to one side of the cancer and the pathologist will report only normal tissue. There are times, too, when needle biopsy will not deliver enough tissue for the pathologist to be positive about the analysis. The needle biopsy can, of course, be repeated if necessary.

How else can a biopsy be done?

Another way of securing tissue is to perform an operation—by cutting through the perineum (the area between the anus and the scrotum) to the prostate. You can thus see the area involved and remove the tissue you want. The operation is halted while the tissue is put through a rapid process called frozen section that enables the pathologist to give an immediate diagnosis. If cancer is present, the surgeon goes on to remove the whole prostate.

Other very sophisticated tests for study of the urinary tracts are available, such as the use of radioactive material injected into the blood to outline the entire kidney substance (renal scan) or to determine the activity of the kidneys (renogram). However, these and many others are used in special cases only and the average man is not likely to encounter them.

8. Operations on the Prostate

> "I'm ashamed to admit it, Doctor, but I'm scared to death. I know I have to have this operation, but I don't know where you're going to cut me open, and I'm afraid I might not come out of the anesthetic. What's more, I hate hospitals."

My patient's fears are understandable. Most modern hospitals are no more than workshops for the physician or surgeon. As in an auto-repair shop, where all the necessary tools, work areas, and machinery are at hand for the mechanic, in a hospital the surgeon has his instruments, operating room, and a wealth of diagnostic and treatment equipment. Ironically, the better the equipment and the more services offered, the more complex and confusing a hospital is likely to be for a patient and his family.

If we had more money, more time, and more personnel, we could undoubtedly make hospitals less frightening to patients. But when hospitals across the country are faced, as they uniformly are, with limited financial resources, they naturally expend those resources on improving medical efficiency rather than in making the surroundings more attractive. As a result, patients often feel needlessly awed and unduly apprehensive. Patients who ask questions in advance of admission, and who demand that their doctors take time to explain procedures, will have a much easier time of it.

The number of hospital admissions in the United States is about thirty million annually. This means that one of every eight persons will find himself hospitalized in any given year. For this reason you may find helpful the following outline of what your experience might be if you had to have prostatic surgery:

What happens when you arrive at the hospital?

Admission generally requires a short interview consisting of routine questions necessary to identify you properly in the hospital's records. Unfortunately, if you are in pain or are apprehensive about a coming operation, you may find this more of a trial than it really is.

How are you prepared for surgery?

Following admission, many preliminary checks are made on you, including blood tests, electrocardiographic tracing, and chest X ray. Also routine may be additional X rays and tests, sometimes taking several days, essential to complete preoperative analysis.

What if you lose blood?

If you are awaiting surgery, your blood will be typed and cross-matched in case a transfusion is needed during or after the operation. The availability of transfusions is crucial to safe surgery. In 1900, an Austrian pathologist discovered that human blood was not all the same and that a patient who received a transfusion of blood unlike his own would suffer dangerous reactions. He found that there were four major groups of blood and that matching the blood of donor and patient made transfusions safe.

Blood was first stored during World War I, but not until 1937 was a major blood bank started, at Cook County Hospital in Chicago. Today whole blood from voluntary donors is routinely stored; refrigerated at proper temperatures, it lasts up to three weeks without significant deterioration. In addition, the red cells and other blood components which can be separated from the fluid portion are stocked for special purposes (such as a clotting agent for cases of hemophilia). Thus, any blood lost during an operation can be quickly replaced by blood-bank supplies.

What about anesthetics—aren't they dangerous?

We have long since passed from the dark ages of anesthesia when only ether and chloroform were available for surgery. Now we have a variety of anesthetics that are safe even for elderly and poor-risk patients.

What does the anesthesiologist do?

The anesthesiologist is not just a doctor who puts you to sleep; he is knowledgeable about respiratory and cardiac functions, and aware of the effects and stresses of the contemplated operation. Together with the urologist, the anesthesiologist will choose the most suitable anesthetic. At times, you may have your choice of either going to sleep or having a spinal (regional) anesthetic.

During the operation, the anesthesiologist regulates the anesthetic, gives a blood transfusion or other fluids as required, and monitors body functions such as heart rate and respiration.

What does prostatectomy consist of?

Though we speak of these operations as removing the prostate, in fact the entire prostate is *not* removed —except in *radical* prostatectomy, which is done only for cancer. The capsule—basically, the compressed outer rim composed of the original prostate—is left behind. The structures removed are the enlarged prostatic *lobes*—that is, overgrown adenomas or nodules which have originated from glands located around the urethra.

Four main techniques are used, and they are named for the area through which the surgeon reaches the prostate gland:

1. Suprapubic prostatectomy—an incision is made *above* the pubic bone.
2. Retropubic prostatectomy—the prostate is removed from *underneath* the pubic bone.
3. Transurethral prostatectomy—instead of making an incision, the surgeon inserts his instruments *through the urethra.*
4. Perineal prostatectomy—an incision is made in the *perineal area* (between the scrotum and the rectum).

Any given urologist is probably skilled in two or three of these techniques and will choose the method best suited to the patient.

What is suprapubic prostatectomy?

This technique is perhaps more frequently used than any other. The surgeon makes an incision in the lower abdomen above the pubic bone, which enables him to make an opening into the bladder. Through this bladder opening he can scoop out the enlarged prostatic lobes with his finger, leaving the capsule of the prostate behind.

One reason this technique is so widely employed is that it has a unique advantage. The surgeon can take a look at the bladder, too, and do any necessary bladder procedures such as removal of a stone, bladder tumor, or diverticulum (an outpouching of the bladder wall).

During the operation, tubes are placed in the bladder and urethra to drain off the urine and to permit washing out of the bladder as necessary. After healing is adequate, removing the tubes is so simple it is done in the patient's room without anesthetic.

Occasionally, when a man has kidney damage because of back pressure from urine retained in a bladder which is not draining properly, this operation is performed in two stages. During the first part, a drainage tube is placed in the bladder. Later (after days or weeks, depending on the patient's condition), when kidney function has been stabilized or restored, the bladder is reopened and the enlarged prostate removed; after final healing, all tubes are taken out.

This two-stage operation, which used to be necessary for complications such as kidney damage, infection, and heart disease, is less common than it used to be. Patients today are coming to surgery before kidney damage has occurred. Also, we can now first treat kidney or bladder infections with modern antibiotics, and then proceed to the one-stage operation. Similarly, while it was formerly felt that a damaged heart would tolerate two smaller procedures better than the full operation, nowadays medical advances can strengthen the heart sufficiently to withstand the one-stage surgery.

What is retropubic prostatectomy?

Here also a lower abdominal incision is made. But instead of approaching the prostate through the bladder, the surgeon makes an opening through the capsule of the prostate *underneath* the pubic bone (hence the name *retro*pubic). The surgeon can then

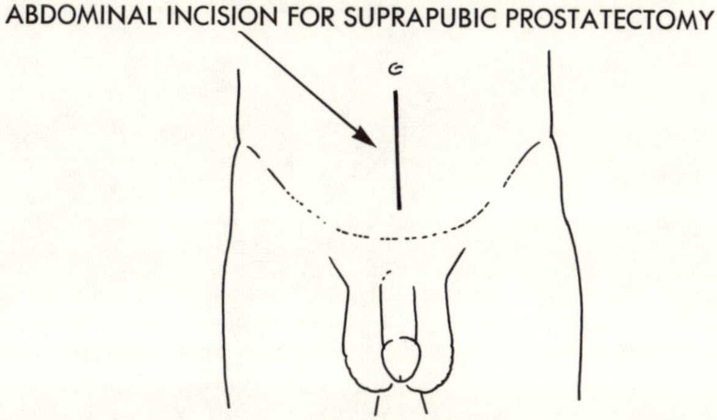

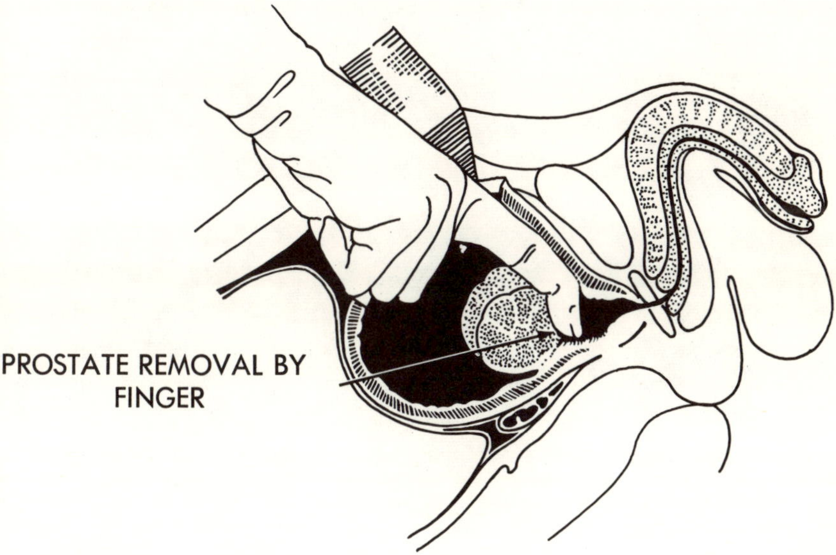

Suprapubic prostatectomy: Probably the most common technique for prostate removal, suprapubic prostatectomy requires an incision through the lower abdomen (*insert*) and bladder. The surgeon simply scoops out the enlarged lobes with his fingers.

remove the enlarged prostatic lobes through the capsule instead of through the bladder (as in suprapubic prostatectomy). Since the bladder is not opened, this type of operation is not suited to any patient with an associated bladder problem. Nevertheless, radical prostatectomy (removal of the prostatic capsule in addition to the enlarged lobes and the seminal vesicles) for early cancer of the prostate is possible by this method.

What is transurethral prostatectomy?

This technique—also called transurethral resection of the prostate, or TURP for short—does not require an abdominal incision. Instead, an ingenious hollow tube (a complex modification of the cystoscope) is inserted through the tip of the penis, via the urethra, to the enlarged prostate. Through this tube the prostate is then shaved or whittled away—much in the same way that a stick of wood is whittled by a knife—with a wire loop activated by an electric current. The loop catches a bit of tissue and cuts it way from the prostate, and by degrees the entire prostate can be removed. Bleeding is controlled by a variation of the same high-frequency electrical current supplied through an electrosurgical unit. As the whittling progresses, fluids can be circulated through the hollow tube to remove the bits of shaved tissue.

After the operation, drainage tubes remain in the bladder for a few days.

This "electrical operation," which has been done since 1931, requires special skills and a highly trained urologist. One disadvantage is that the urethra is a slender tube and cannot be stretched too much; the cystoscopelike instrument must therefore also be narrow, and it provides limited access to the prostate. However, this method is used everywhere in the world with great safety and success.

While this transurethral procedure appeals to patients because there is no external incision, and because it requires a shorter hospital stay and convalescence, it should not be regarded as a minor operation. It is as much of an operation as any other technique and carries many of the same surgical risks.

The transurethral operation is ideally suited for a prostate gland which has not yet enlarged too much. A huge prostatic enlargement calls for an "open" operation—that is, with an incision—to remove the sizable amounts of tissue. Shaving away an enormously overgrown gland would keep the patient on the operating table too long and cause other technical problems.

What is perineal prostatectomy?

A perineal approach to the prostate is not used as frequently as the above methods because of two special risks: there are greater dangers that a man will lose his sexual ability and that he will lose urinary control than with any of the other techniques.

Here an incision must be made in front of the rectum—in the space just behind the scrotum. When the surgeon cuts into this area, so richly supplied with nerves, it is difficult not to damage or sever nerves controlling sexual and urinary mechanisms.

Just as a doctor can feel the prostate by inserting a

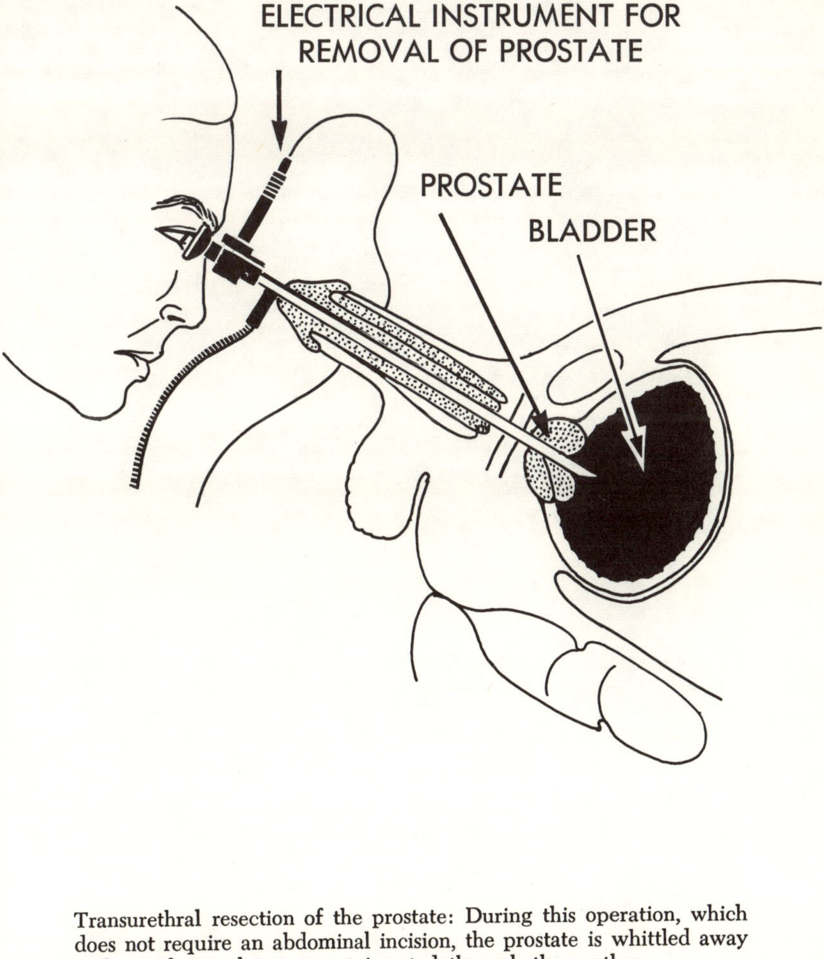

Transurethral resection of the prostate: During this operation, which does not require an abdominal incision, the prostate is whittled away with an electrical instrument inserted through the urethra.

finger into the rectum, the surgeon gets to the gland by making an incision in the perineal area. He then pushes back the rectal wall, cuts through the capsule wall, and removes the prostatic lobes through the capsule.

Historically, this is the oldest of the operations used for prostatectomy, for a bladder stone was removed through this type of incision some three centuries before Christ. Though naturally greatly refined in our own time, it is not as commonly used as the other procedures. It is, however, especially useful for men who require radical prostatectomy for a cancer which has not yet begun to spread.

What is cryosurgery of the prostate?

Within the last decade, we have learned to destroy the prostate through freezing. Liquid nitrogen, at minus 196 degrees centigrade, flows through a metal probe inserted through the urethra to the prostate and kills the prostatic tissue by lowering its temperature to minus 40 degrees centigrade. The dead tissue subsequently falls away and is voided with the urine.

Although it sounds ingenious, this method has not become very popular because it is a "blind" operation —the urologist cannot see the tissue he is freezing. Another disadvantage is that the dead tissue does not come away at once; it sloughs off or rots away over a period of weeks and can cause new urinary blockage —the condition which the operation was done to overcome. Nevertheless, cryosurgery is valuable in certain cases, for example, for an older man in poor health who might not readily withstand the more conventional techniques.

What happens after the operation is finished?

Following any operation, the patient is taken from the operating suite to the recovery room. Here experienced nurses can monitor him for changes in his heartbeat and breathing until the anesthetic has worn off. Because the recovery room is always located on the operating-suite floor, the anesthesiologist can check the patient at intervals and the surgeon can drop by to satisfy himself that all is going well, that drainage tubes are functioning properly, and that there is no excessive bleeding.

Most men take great comfort in knowing that they will receive this careful, highly technical attention before being returned to their room. It is reassuring to know that any slight postoperative change will be immediately noted and that all the equipment for further treatment is right at hand. As a result, patients have lost their fear of dying *after* the operation, as used to be common some time ago.

Are there likely to be any postoperative complications?

Postoperative complications are possible, but fortunately infrequent. *Any* type of surgery can be followed, for example, by hemorrhage or infection or pneumonia; and, knowing this, the urologist surrounds his patient with every known medical protective device. He will have blood available for transfusion, give appropriate "miracle" antibiotics to avoid or combat infection, and constantly monitor the heart for any cardiac emergency. These multiple measures will usually obviate or overcome postoperative troubles.

There are, however, two other difficulties that may follow any type of prostatic operation: incontinence (loss of urinary control), and stricture or contracture (urinary blockage). Fortunately, neither one happens frequently.

How is incontinence caused?

Since the prostate lies just between two urinary control muscles, or sphincters—the internal one at the bladder outlet, and the external one in the urethra—surgery to the prostate can injure these muscles. Damage to the internal sphincter is of no importance and can be completely disregarded. It is injury to the external sphincter which can make a man incontinent.

In those few cases in which incontinence occurs postoperatively, it is usually temporary. This embarrassing wetting requires no treatment, and within a few weeks to a couple of months the muscle readjusts and the patient regains complete control.

More permanent incontinence does occur occasionally, especially after transurethral prostatectomy, and this is of course very distressing. Should it happen, we instruct the patient in exercises which often successfully strengthen the sphincter. If they don't work, he may have to wear a penis clamp or collecting device. Operations to repair the injured muscle are notoriously ineffective, though a few have been successful.

What causes urinary blockage?

After prostatic surgery, scar tissue can form a ring either at the bladder exit, where it is called contracture, or in the urethra, where it is called stricture. In either case, it causes the same symptoms as the original enlargement of the prostate (a slow urinary stream and perhaps frequency of urination). Fortunately, this complication is not serious and can be overcome by stretching the narrowed area with dilating instruments, an office procedure. Rarely, the urologist may actually have to make a cut through the contracting ring of scar tissue.

Will prostatic surgery affect your sex life?

Under ordinary circumstances, prostate removal—whether transurethral, retropubic, or suprapubic—should not cause any reduction in the sexual ability of any man. In most cases, however, men will no longer ejaculate externally. This is because anatomic changes after removal of the prostate cause the semen to go backward into the bladder. But erection and orgasm are unchanged, and all the feelings and emotions of climax are the same as before the operation.

I always explain to a patient about to undergo a prostatic operation that sexually he will be no better and no worse; the only difference will be an inability to father any more children because of the absence of an emission. Since most men who require these operations are past the age when they will want children, this causes no hardship. Only in the rare instance of a younger man who still desires children is lack of emission a problem.

There is a totally different sexual picture, however, when the perineal prostatic operation is done. The incision and dissection used in this surgical method routinely cut across certain nerves affecting erection, so that in many cases there is some or even total impotence.

Does having a prostatectomy mean you won't ever have prostatic trouble again?

As I explained earlier, in none of the routine operations named above is the *entire* prostate removed, only the enlarged lobes. Since the prostatic capsule is left behind, regrowth of obstructing tissue is possible. A man may even develop cancer of the prostate at some later date. Renewed prostatic growth or development of cancer following prostatectomy is infrequent, but it does happen. It is almost like having tonsils regrow after they have been removed.

Note: Readers interested in a more technical explanation of urogenital surgical procedures might wish to consult the step-by-step description in my illustrated *Atlas of Urologic Surgery,* published by Appleton-Century-Crofts, New York.

9. Especially for Women—Sexual Problems in Your Mate

They were both young—a recently married couple—and they were both at swords' points. Why wasn't this early marriage succeeding? Was this sweet young lady such a nag and termagant? Was this good-looking, seemingly fine adult male a real dud? It took a lot of probing to secure a true picture from the two reluctant-to-speak people. The cause was sexual, the wife not sufficiently mature and knowledgeable to comprehend her husband's problem.

For women it is almost impossible to realize—even imagine—the embarrasment, chagrin, worry, and despair a man feels when he fails to perform adequately in sexual contact. An erect penis is such a strong symbol of maleness that a man unable to secure a satisfactory erection feels that his adequacy as a total man comes into question.

In a man who feels secure and loved, this might produce only mild anxiety. In a man under any sort of stress–on the job, socially, in his marriage–it can be bitterly devastating.

In the next chapter, I try to indicate the many causes of impotence; and I feel strongly that, while a relationship can benefit by a woman's understanding of *all* the urogenital problems her mate might face, it is impotence that should most concern a woman. It is a rare marriage that does not have to face impotence at one time or another–either as a temporary phenomenon, as a recurrent one, or as a chronic or prolonged problem. Moreover, impotence is not predictable. It can occur on a wedding night or at a primary encounter, but it can also occur after many years of a successful sexual relationship. How a woman reacts at such times can be vital not only to her mate's happiness but to the future course of the relationship itself.

Why is it up to a woman?

A wise woman realizes that while she herself will have a variety of reactions to sexual activity, she does not have to perform the kind of physical alteration equivalent to an erection. She can, of course, be more than cooperative in sex, but she can also fake it a bit if she feels tired or unenthusiastic at any time. Her mate has no such recourse–he must produce an erection or intercourse is impossible. Thus the pressure is always on him.

How can a woman help?

In the complete circuit of psychic stimulation, male hormone (testosterone) action, electrical nerve stimulation, and blood engorgement of the erectile tissue, things may go awry at any point. An intelligent woman will therefore be aware of, and quick to sympathize with, any circumstances that adversely affect her mate's sexual performance.

Since poor erections can be caused by remediable conditions such as prostatitis or other ailments, adequate medical care should concern both partners. A wife should also know whether her husband is suffering from some medical problem (such as diabetes or arteriosclerosis) or whether he is taking medication (some high-blood-pressure tablets and some tranquilizers) which causes impotence.

Yet, most impotence is not physical in origin or induced by medication or drugs. Most of it is psychological—and for this reason the support and sympathy of the woman are crucial.

What if the cause is psychological?

Criticism, caustic remarks, or any other sort of intimation that the wife is disappointed is only going to increase a man's sense of failure and aggravate the physical problem.

And this is not simply a bedroom matter. If a man is impotent because he has lost his job, it is not going to help matters any if his wife is sympathetic in bed because he can't get an erection but berates him at other times for failing to support the family. Nor is a woman who pretends great passivity during intercourse going to make her husband feel less emasculated if she nags at him or bosses him all the rest of the time.

So a woman who is affirmative in her love, who does not see impotence as an affront to herself or as a failure in her husband, can do much to assuage the anguish and self-doubt in her mate.

What specific action can a woman take?

When her husband is impotent a woman can remind herself of how dramatically she affects his sexual response. If in coping with children or other duties she has let herself go, she no longer bothers to comb her hair or look attractive, she might reconsider whether paying more attention to herself might not make a difference; improving her physical appearance might not only entice her husband, but make *her* feel sexier and more desirable, too.

Perhaps it might be time to examine whether the couple has fallen into the rut of disregarding each other's idiosyncrasies. Does she do something that turns off her mate—such as wearing pin curlers to bed—something she might have been careful to avoid in the early days of the relationship, but which has turned into a careless habit after long familiarity? Sometimes, unsuspected and unnoticed by the woman, a trivial action or routine may be so annoying or distasteful to a man that he becomes sexually inhibited. Perhaps, too, the common courtesies have been replaced by demands, or an attitude of taking everything for granted.

Self-study should be part of every woman's role as a sexual mate. Does she act solely as a compliant, almost inert individual in sex, or does she participate enthusiastically? Does she play an equal role in courting, or does she leave all decisions about when to have sex to her husband?

Impotence, then, may be a condition of a man, but among its many causes and ramifications may be some attributable to a woman or to the condition of a relationship. A sympathetic, cooperative approach by the woman, together with a specific study of her role, may solve *his* problem!

10. Impotence

> "I'm desperate, Doctor, because suddenly I can't get an erection. I can't eat, sleep, or work—my marriage is in danger. You've got to help me!"

The inability to perform sexually and the consequent fear that he is no longer a man is perhaps the most serious blow a man's ego can receive. Though impotence is the butt of many jokes, its effects are tragic. If it comes on abruptly, particularly in a young man, he can suffer devastating unhappiness; a truly severe upheaval can even lead to suicide.

How common is impotence?

Despite everything written about sex in modern times, there are virtually no statistics about impotence. We don't know how many men suffer from this problem or at what ages it is most common. No one can really say, because men don't like to talk about it, and when they do it's hard to tell if they are being entirely truthful.

Temporary impotence is undoubtedly frequent but unimportant since it disappears of its own accord. Often it is simply due to tension or exhaustion rather than to any serious mental or physical defect.

Isolated instances of impotence are probably also very common. For instance, an overly eager man, beset with anxiety and desire on his honeymoon night, may fail utterly in his attempt at coitus, particularly if he has had no prior sexual experience.

Such isolated and temporary examples of impotence probably occur in the lives of most men but they are nothing to worry about.

Impotence, as we will deal with it here, is of the type sufficiently *frequent* or *persistent* to affect a man's happiness.

What is impotence?

Frankly, we have no way of objectively measuring impotence—it can only be assessed subjectively by the man who suffers from it. Though many things in medicine are subjective, we usually find ways of measuring them; pain, for instance, is purely subjective, yet we can gauge its intensity as well as the effectiveness of any particular pain-killer on any particular individual. However, we are not yet privileged except under very special artificial and experimental circumstances to measure a couple's sexual performance or to assess the man's subjective evaluation.

Our best medical definition therefore is that potency means the ability to achieve and sustain erection and successfully conclude the act of coitus. Thus an erection firm enough for vaginal penetration and sustained enough to lead to orgasm would constitute adequate potency. Conversely, a weak erection, premature ejaculation, or an erection that cannot be maintained until the man or woman secures orgasm would constitute varying degrees of impotence.

Why is it so difficult to define impotence?

Impotence is complicated because it involves two people. For example, in some premature ejaculations, a man reaches orgasm before he wants to. In other cases, ejaculatory orgasm may be satisfactory for the man but disappointing to his partner. And in some cases, neither will be satisfied. Despite a firm erection, a man is impotent in all these cases because his ejaculation has come too early, with consequent loss of erection, to constitute a fully satisfactory sexual experience for *both* partners.

Isn't sex frequency a measure of potency?

No. Having successful sexual intercourse often or regularly is not truly a measure of adequate potency because frequency depends on many factors not involved in sex; and since it also depends on mutual agreement, it is complicated by the needs and desires of a man's partner as well as his own.

Sex frequency is often connected with relaxation, and freedom from strains and tensions. A couple away on vacation will ordinarily indulge in more sex than at home. Similarly, because of external pressures, many men, as they get older and achieve more status in society or more responsibility in business, may find themselves less interested in sex. Although they may chalk this up to advancing age, the real reason may be in their increasing strains and responsibilities.

Isn't age a factor?

To some extent, yes. We know that the height of male sexual ability is generally in a man's early twenties and that it slowly tapers off from that time on, with a more abrupt decline occurring in the sixth decade of life. Nevertheless, as I explain in Chapter 12, men vary in how long they retain sexual interest and ability.

Why is it so hard to set standards of "normal" potency?

An immensely complicating factor is libido, or sexual *drive* or *desire*, which is greatly influenced by innumerable factors such as background, education, experiences, and motivation in life and goals. For example, a priest may remain potent, but his libido is generally sublimated because he trains himself to play down and deny instinctive sexual drives and to direct these energies into intense concern for others. Likewise, some men are molded by motivation toward a specific goal so that sex becomes secondary. A man intent on becoming a millionaire might put all his energy into making money; his sexual drive might very well be diminished, but he continues to be potent. A scientist working day and night in intense research can be so absorbed in his work that his sexual drives are minimal, but he, too, remains potent. Libido and potency thus are not equivalent terms. The greatly troubled man is the one who retains his desire for intercourse (libido) and is unable to carry it through to orgasmic fulfillment (potency).

Then what does "oversexed" or "undersexed" mean?

These terms are confusing. Frequency of intercourse varies in different people, just as people vary in height, size, or appetite for food. A man may fear he is oversexed or undersexed because he has greater or lesser sexual drive than his sexual partner. But comparison is made only with that one partner. With another person, whose sexual needs approach his own, he would be normally sexed. People vary so much in their sexual appetites and habits that setting standards for "normal" is impossible.

Does penis size affect potency?

I am often asked, "Doctor, I think my penis is too small; what do you think?"

The length and width of the penis—whether erect or not erect—varies from man to man and is no more important than the length of his nose, depth of forehead, or size and spacing of his eyes. It is not the size of an erect penis which makes for adequate sexual response—in either men or women. A woman's vagina distends only for the size of the penis which is inserted, so the dimensions of the penis make no difference to either partner. Moreover, the involuntary muscular contractions which occur in female orgasm are in the outer one-third of the vagina—and even the smallest erect penis goes beyond this depth. Indeed, the heavy thrusting of a very large penis could even be so uncomfortable as to lessen a woman's sexual feelings.

Sexual satisfaction varies from one woman to another. Add to this fact that a woman may be conditioned by gossip and misinformation—she may believe that a penis must be a certain size before she can be satisfied. Such a woman will have to be reconditioned to the truth that a smaller or larger penis can produce equal satisfaction.

The same conditioning can be true of a man. A man who believes the myths about a large penis may ruin his sexual enjoyment by unnecessary anxiety and feelings of inferiority. The man is greatly mistaken if he believes that a small penis makes him a poor lover. Female sexual response is a combination of physical, psychological, and emotional aspects; and so lovemaking and orgasm involve factors other than the size of the penis.

What causes impotence?

Broadly speaking, there are two forms of impotence: one from physical causes, the other from psychological difficulties. On occasion, the two may be mixed. For instance, a man may have a physical abnormality which prevents adequate erection; yet his problem may be compounded because his abnormality makes him feel inferior.

Which type of impotence is most common?

Most well-informed estimates show that nine-tenths of all cases of impotence are based on psychological or emotional causes. Proof of this is that the more intellectual or cultured a man is, the greater are his chances of suffering from impotence. The more basic or instinctive the individual, the less likely he is to have difficulty with erections. Our natural sexual impulses are easily and dramatically affected by our civilized layers and practices.

Sexual intercourse consists of several stages: mental and emotional sexual drive which leads to arousal; physical genital interaction which terminates in orgasm (and ejaculation in the male); and finally resolution (with disappearance of erection in the man). As difficulties may occur anywhere along this chain to abort the totality of the sex act, there can be many facets and nuances of impotence.

PHYSICAL CAUSES

What are common physical causes of impotence?

Temporary and permanent physical causes include birth defects, certain diseases (such as Peyronie's disease, diabetes, or diseases of the nervous system), hormone deficiencies, malnutrition, and certain injuries and operations. Some urinary-tract and prostate problems can also result in impotence; in fact, severe illness of any sort can cause temporary loss of potency. Common (but often unrecognized) sources of trouble are drugs and alcohol, and perhaps certain chemicals. Occasionally a rare disorder, such as Leriche's syndrome or priapism, will cause a man to be impotent.

Can birth defects be cured?

The most obvious birth defects are failure of the penis or other sexual organs to develop, and sometimes this failure, as described in Chapter 1, can be treated or cured.

Other abnormalities, such as a large water sac in the scrotum which conceals the penis, are less well-known. Many of these can also often be corrected by surgery.

Which diseases of the nervous system cause impotence?

Injury to the spinal cord, pressure on the spinal cord by a herniated disc, multiple sclerosis, or other general nerve ailments such as syphilis may make a man unable to have erections. In a form of epilepsy, that involving the temporal lobe of the brain, impotence is an outstanding symptom.

What is Peyronie's disease?

In this ailment, the cause of which is unknown, scar tissue develops in the erectile portions of the penis.

This scar tissue produces curvature on erection, often making it impossible to insert the penis into the vagina.

Can diabetes cause impotence?

Poor erections are not uncommon in diabetic men; this is especially so when the diabetes is not well controlled and is of long standing. The exact mechanism of this impotence is not certain, but it may be due to minimal and undetectable nerve damage or to some hormonal imbalance. (Insulin, a hormone, is deficient in diabetics, and so the entire hormonal mechanism may be thrown out of kilter.) Certainly, potency is better if the diabetes is under good control. Men whose diabetes started in childhood or adolescence are more frequently impotent.

Which other hormone deficiencies cause impotence?

Thyroid underfunction (hypothyroidism) can cause impotence, but this can usually be corrected by giving thyroid hormone pills.

Lack of sufficient male sex hormone can also make an erection impossible. This is true of men whose testicles underfunction or malfunction because of birth defects; their disorder is known as hypogonadism and is associated with other physical features. Eunuchs and youngsters castrated because of injury before puberty are usually incapable of erection. In most cases of this type, artificial male sex hormones can be administered as a substitute for testicular function, thus restoring potency, but such individuals are nevertheless sterile.

What is Leriche's syndrome?

This disease is characterized by a reduction in blood flow. Its outstanding symptom is inability to walk any appreciable distance because of poor blood circulation to the legs—but the sex organs are also deprived of their necessary blood supply, so an erection is impossible. Surgical treatment is at times successful in restoring proper blood supply to both the pelvis and the legs. With improvement in blood circulation, potency returns.

What is priapism?

Oddly enough, this condition is named after the Greek god of fertility and reproduction, Priapus. There is persistent, prolonged, and painful erection which may last for days, even weeks. Sometimes it comes on from sexual excitation, but at other times its cause is unknown. Priapism can also be caused by sickle-cell anemia, by leukemia, or by cancer deposits in the penis.

The most successful treatment is surgery within thirty-six hours after the priapism begins; the operation forms a new channel from the rodlike structure in the rigid penis to the veins of the pelvis to allow outflow of entrapped blood.

This abnormal sustained erection, however, is frequently followed by permanent impotence, even when early treatment or surgery is successful in securing a reduction in the priapism.

What kind of urinary problems decrease potency?

Urinary-tract disorders such as stricture of the urethra, inflammation of the bladder, and prostatitis may decrease potency.

Premature ejaculation can occur with lower urinary-tract ailments and is often brought on by inflammation in the urethra and verumontanum, which is associated with prostatitis. Since the prostate and urinary channels play an important role in ejaculation, any inflammation in this supersensitive region can trigger premature ejaculation. This type of problem is readily diagnosed and treated once pus cells are found in the fluid secured from a tender, boggy prostate.

Which drugs or chemicals affect potency?

"Hard" drugs, such as heroin, and some tranquilizers frequently reduce potency. Narcotics or sedatives, such as barbiturates, morphine derivatives, or alcohol, can cause impotence more often than is recognized. Even cigarette smoking has been known to reduce potency.

However, often the emotional needs that bring on a drug or alcohol habit also make the impotence more pronounced.

Some of our newer drugs and chemicals—used in food, or around the house or as medicinals—may have side effects on potency. Usually, there is no way to tell whether a new drug produces such side effects until the product has been used long enough for reactions to be reported to medical authorities: any new product may have a yet unknown influence on sexual potency.

What about aphrodisiacs?

No drug acts as a true aphrodisiac, nor is any particular food or vitamin known to improve male potency (although malnutrition can cause impotence). Stories of such improvement—which is supposed to come from items ranging from raw eggs to raw oysters to watermelon seeds—are, unfortunately, old wives' tales. Improvement, if any, is purely psychological—the man convinces himself in advance that the raw eggs or other foods are going to perform wonders.

Will surgery to a man's sexual organs make him impotent?

This depends on the surgery.

The most common types of operations performed on the prostate, for example, usually do not cause impotence (see Chapter 8).

Males who must have both testicles removed will usually not be able to have erections if this operation is done *before* puberty. However, as explained in Chapter 1, when testicular loss occurs *after* puberty, satisfactory erection and intercourse are possible in some cases because habit patterns have been formed and because male sex hormone is not truly essential for erection in adult men.

Other types of urogenital surgery—to correct birth defects or injuries, or surgery necessitated by disease—are rarer and unlikely to be experienced by the average man. An illustration might be the man who suffers a pelvic fracture. If this accident injures the urethra and deep pelvic nerves, impotence often results, either from the injury or from the injury plus the surgery necessary to repair the urethra. This is a melancholy sequel to a pelvic fracture because damaged pelvic nerves cannot be repaired or replaced.

What other injuries can cause impotence?

Damage to the perineum (the area between the rectum and scrotum), such as in a straddle accident, may cause impotence. Straddle injuries often occur in young boys, for example, who walk along the top of a fence, lose their balance, and land on top of the fence, with a picket impaling the perineum.

PSYCHOLOGICAL CAUSES

How can a man tell if his impotence is psychologically caused?

Emotional or psychological causes of impairment of potency are varied and more frequent than physical causes. Most men, however, cannot admit to themselves that they have psychological troubles, so they prefer to believe the cause is physical. In addition, it may be difficult for a man to recognize that his problem is emotional because its origins may go back to his childhood and be buried in his unconscious mind.

It is a clue that impotence is psychological when a man can get an erection under one set of circumstances yet not in another. A good example is the man who thinks he is impotent yet has an early-morning erection. Obviously his physical mechanisms are functioning well but some mental block exists. Another illustration is the man who can secure erections by fantasy or masturbation but not by sexual contact. Again, no anatomic or physical basis exists for the lack of potency.

How can the unconscious mind cause impotence?

If a boy was punished for masturbating—or even if he was not punished but was aware that his parents disapproved of the practice—he could grow up linking sex with fear of punishment. Even when he reached adulthood and tried to enjoy sex, he could still carry these fears in his unconscious mind and they could hold him back. Likewise, a child terrorized by stories that masturbation would damage his later sexual ability could be unaware of carrying this specter of damage into adulthood even if his conscious mind told him it was nonsense.

Does masturbation affect potency?

Masturbation is almost universal and has no detrimental effect on a man's sex life. Even very frequent masturbation won't produce any important organic disturbance of any kind. Unfortunately, however, sex education is so poor in our schools that it is hard for boys to grow up without picking up distorted notions from parents and playmates. Such inadequate or faulty sex education—not masturbation itself—produces many of the sexual inhibitions later in life.

Is fear of masturbation the only childhood experience that can cause impotence?

Not by any means—it just happens to be one of the most common. There simply isn't enough space here to detail the enormously long list of distorted views (about male and female anatomy; about fears that sex is dirty or cruel; illogical notions of how one or the other partner should react; and so forth) that have been known to cause impotence in men (and frigidity in women). Problems are often compounded because both the men and the women are misinformed and burdened with irrational phobias.

Lack of correct information is so common that young couples often have difficulty adjusting to each other. Emotional factors resulting from misinformation together with inexperience, ineptness, or fear of hurting his partner may make a man's early sex experience disastrous. This can then progress from an initial potency failure to a full-blown sexual problem.

Young people whose chief difficulty is merely ignorance can sometimes become more sure of themselves by consulting informational books; if the problems are more deep-seated, professional guidance (by the family physician, perhaps, or the marriage counselor) may be required to avert this type of tragedy.

Is misinformation the chief childhood influence on impotence?

It is not so much misinformation but the composite of childhood experiences which determine how a particular child will view himself and the world about him in adult life. This is not a question of facts but of feelings. For instance, psychiatrists stress that a man's very strong attachments to his mother may influence his behavior (including sexual activity) with other women; because he identifies other women with his mother, he views—consciously or unconsciously—sexual union as incest and is thus unable to go through with the sex act.

Similarly, children who have come from broken homes, or have had abusive or painful backgrounds, often unconsciously carry into adulthood distorted views about women, sex, or family life that can adversely affect their sexual capabilities.

Is psychological impotence a sign of some deep mental problem?

Although impotence may be one of many symptoms of a severe emotional problem (a psychiatrist might term this "celibacy complex"), it is important to distinguish between grave mental problems which require psychiatric help and those caused by a temporary stress situation in which a man happens to find himself.

Sometimes a man is impotent at home and potent in an extramarital experience: here it is clear we are dealing with a man who has neither a physical disability nor any deep or radical psychological ailment. Rather we have a victim of marital boredom or tension. This situation might be resolved through mutual understanding and cooperation with his wife. In other cases the impotence can be traced to a nonresponsive or nagging wife, and in these cases, she rather than her husband requires counseling or treatment.

If a man's sexual drive is much stronger than his wife's, he may avoid the frustration and resentment of being refused by ceasing to make advances. Such sexual repression, if practiced long enough, may result in complete impotence.

Is the problem always related to sex?

No. Simple emotional difficulties that have nothing to do with sex, such as anxiety over some everyday matter, may also seriously inhibit potency.

What are the most common kinds of problem?

From my own files, here are brief case histories that illustrate psychological causes of impotence. As these are fairly typical, some readers may find circumstances similar to their own:

Case I: A twenty-one-year-old youth had had an operation in early childhood for a birth defect of the penis; this defect had been successfully repaired so that now he was quite normal physically. Nevertheless, several times a year he required treatment (stretching of the urethra) to make sure that the urinary passageway remained wide open.

He had had no trouble in early sexual encounters and coitus. But then, when he was called up for the draft and rejected on physical grounds because of the urethral narrowing, he suddenly became impotent.

Subconsciously he felt that if the Army thought he was "not enough of a man" to accept him, then the symbol of his maleness, an erect penis, had no valid grounds; so subconsciously the stimulus for erection disappeared. Once I had reassured him that he had been rejected solely because his necessary periodic treatment might not be available under field conditons, his problem cleared up.

In this instance, a physical deformity which had actually been corrected masked a psychological cause of impotence.

Case II: A thirty-two-year-old man who had never had a sexual experience married—only to discover he was impotent. He had such fear of being unable to satisfy his wife that he did not even attempt intercourse. I spent many hours talking to him, reassuring him, before he gained enough confidence to secure an effective erection. Having overcome this initial fear and self-doubt, he then had no problem with sex.

Case III: A fifty-six-year-old man came to me because he had suddenly become impotent after thirty years of satisfactory marital relations. When I questioned him I learned that he had lost his job after many years of service, and he was frightened that he might not be able to find another at his age.

For several sessions we discussed how his fear of being unable to earn a living was to him the equivalent of no longer being head of the household and therefore no longer a "man." As a result, the loss of his job culminated in the loss of his symbol of maleness, an erection. Realizing the interrelationship of the two ideas helped, and when he found another job his problem was completely eliminated.

CASE IV: A thirty-eight-year-old man who had been having poor erections for several years finally was unable to have any erection at all. Though I examined him, I could find no organic problem, so I questioned him about his private life.

He told me his wife was a career woman who had always earned a good salary but that recently her earnings had topped his; in addition, through the ten years of their marriage, she had managed home finances and made all family decisions.

Here, then, was a husband who had gradually given up his male role to his wife; now relinquishing this role included relinquishing his potency, too. We had to have many conferences; but luckily his wife was a perceptive woman who was willing to reverse her own dominating status to help her husband overcome his difficulty.

CASE V: A forty-year-old handsome dentist with an attractive wife and two children fathered in the early years of their marriage had been impotent for a long time. He had been equally unsuccessful in his attempts at extramarital affairs. Yet I could find no physical abnormalities when I examined him.

However, in talking to him I discovered that he daydreamed a great deal and that he had some rather odd habits, such as always sitting in a chair in the corner of whatever room he was in and refusing to go to bed at night unless he wore a special old bathrobe. I referred him to a psychiatrist who diagnosed him as a schizophrenic who had reverted to a narcissistic level. In simple terms, the man was wrapped up in himself and withdrawn; obviously the lack of potency was a sign of a rather serious mental disorder.

From these examples you can see that psychological impotence can stem from either simple and easily correctable causes or from very serious emotional disturbances.

In choosing these cases, I do not mean to imply that they represent the only reasons for impotence; they do, however, provide general guidelines to the underlying anxieties I see most frequently in my practice. What is common to them all is a loss of self-esteem, a fear that one is not virile enough.

When that fear settles unreasonably on a physical part of the body, it need not be so obvious or dramatic as with the boy who had had an operation on his penis; some of my younger patients have been emotionally upset over biceps muscles they thought were too small or even by having a simple case of acne.

Similarly, a man doesn't need a domineering wife to feel deprived of his manhood; he can experience similar despair if he feels he is competing unsuccessfully with his father, his brother, or some business associate.

And loss of employment is only one of many losses which can devastate a man almost overnight; a financial reversal, the death of a friend, the deprivation of status (as through retirement), a teen-age son leaving home or getting into trouble—all these and many more are emotional blows that can be reflected in a man's body so as to affect adversely his sexual life.

TREATMENT

Since impotence manifests itself in varying degrees of severity and since its causes range from simple physical problems or mild anxiety to grave mental disorders, it is obvious that treatment cannot be listed with a few pat suggestions. Treatment must be tailored for each individual, and all I can do here is to give an idea of the way in which I might proceed in evaluating a specific case.

What does a doctor do when a man consults him for impotence?

I find it most unfortunate that most of my patients cannot immediately reveal to me the extent of their distress. Usually they are so conditioned to treat impotence as a grim joke on themselves that they try to make light of it or even to poke fun at themselves and their own plight. Often it takes awhile for me to put my patients at their ease and convince them that I am sympathetic, will not pass judgment on their sexual inabilities, and am willing to listen and to help.

Since my job is to seek the cause of the impotence, the patient's history is very important to me; I must probe his intimate life and press for answers even if the man finds it embarrassing to reveal sexual details. Often patients are tempted to be evasive or less than honest, and I must repeat my assurances that any disclosures to me will be kept in confidence.

Whenever possible, I interview the wife as well, because she will usually be less inhibited in discussing her husband's problem and because it gives me a chance to size her up, too, to find out whether her attitudes might be contributing to her husband's difficulty.

How is the specific cause diagnosed?

The prime question is whether the impotence is physically or emotionally based. Distinguishing between them is not always easy.

If there *is* a physical ailment, such as one of those outlined earlier in this chapter, medication or even surgery may be necessary (see the chapters on diseases and prostatic surgery). Yet many diagnostic tests may have to be done before such a conclusion can be reached and proper treatment begun. Sometimes consultation with other specialists, such as endocrinologists, may be necessary.

If the problem is psychological, I may still have to spend a lot of time before definitely excluding all the possible physical factors. Sometimes, as in the case of the boy who had a physical defect of his penis (page 141), dispensing with a physical problem reveals a deeper emotional one, or an emotional one may arise later. And then treatment in these cases varies enormously. Sometimes a seemingly complex psychological problem vanishes after only a short discussion in which the man becomes aware of his underlying anxieties. In other cases, endless sessions are necessary because it takes longer to discover the underlying tensions or because finding them does not always lead immediately to ways of coping with them.

Who should treat impotence?

If I feel a patient has a good rapport with his family doctor, I may refer the patient to him or work in conjunction with him. In other instances when I feel I can help, I may treat the patient myself. In still other cases, I feel it best to work with a psychiatrist.

What kind of treatment is used?

Obviously, this is a very broad subject, because the treatment must deal with the specific cause and the causes are so varied. Loss of male potency is so complex to treat adequately that no hard and fast rules can apply, and a treatment program must be thought out for each individual. Even when I have ruled out all physical factors, the range of emotionally significant possibilities to be considered can be seen in my discussion of psychological causes above and especially in the case histories on pages 141–144.

From my own experience, however, I have developed two very strong opinions concerning treatment:

First, I believe that a cooperative sexual partner is of paramount importance. A wife must be sympathetic, understanding, and willing to help her husband. Her attitude predicts the eventual outcome: if the wife is uninterested or antagonistic, or if she belittles her husband, it is most unlikely that the man will regain his sexual potency.

Second, I am very much against giving testosterone (male sex hormone) except in a few special cases. There is a use for this hormone in some patients with testicular failure at puberty, but I think it is unwise to assume that testicular function declines with age and that a shot of testosterone is going to cure impotence. As described in Chapter 12, even in very advanced age sexual activity is not only possible but common. The decline of sexual activity with age in many men may therefore be dependent on life style, social pressures, and other factors rather than any hormone deficiency.

What bothers me most about injections of testosterone is that they carry a potential danger. We know that hidden in the depths of the prostate there may be a latent group of cancer cells which ordinarily would not produce any trouble but which can do so when they are stimulated by testosterone injections. This kind of treatment therefore seems to me to carry too high a risk to be justified.

What if all treatment fails?

Urologists can resort to a relatively new operation. Many animals have a bone in the penis: the squirrel has only a tiny sliver, while the walrus has a penis bone over one foot long and more than six inches in circumference. Such a bone is nature's substitution in animals with little erectile tissue. It is only natural therefore that urologists thought of implanting a similar stiff object in a human penis to aid erection.

Cartilage and bone were used first; but cartilage turned out to curl because it was too soft, and bone dissolved. Silicone, which is inert, unbreakable, and resilient, was subsequently introduced and has been used successfully.

A rod of silicone is placed between the two corpora of the penis and enclosed under the fibrous envelope and skin. The silicone rod is placed so that the penis hangs unobtrusively at rest; yet at times of coitus, the penis is rigid enough to be lifted to insert into and deeply penetrate the vagina. The results are most rewarding, but patients must be carefully chosen for this operation. It cannot be indiscriminately suggested for any and all patients who complain of impotence; for a patient with a deep psychological problem—which includes impotence as one symptom—will still have his emotional difficulty after the operation and will still be dissatisfied.

Not all urologists are familiar with and experienced in this new operative technique, which demands considerable attention to detail and which has complications of its own. Thus if the operation is resorted to, an experienced urologic surgeon must be chosen.

11. Is There a Male Menopause?

"I'm worried about Richard," the wife of a patient told me. "He's always been jolly and contented. Now he's moody and disjointed, he has lost his ambition and is worried about his job. He's even losing his sex ability. Is he having a change of life, like a woman, at his age of forty-nine?"

"Strictly speaking," I said, "the answer is no, but . . ."

What is menopause?

Abrupt physical change occurs in a middle-aged woman. Quite suddenly her ovaries stop producing hormones (estrogens) and her menstruation—visible proof of childbearing ability—ceases. Often she becomes irritable and depressed.

Does a man go through menopause?

Many men, on reaching their late forties or early fifties, have emotional problems similar to those of a woman going through "change of life." But a middle-aged man does not have any telltale physical sign. Though his testosterone progressively declines, it never reaches zero level, as does a woman's estrogen. A man does lose some sexual energy in addition to other physical capabilities as the years pass, but his reproductive ability doesn't disappear as does a woman's. So these feelings of inadequacy, depression, and other emotions which remind us of the female menopause are not strictly comparable.

Then what is the male menopause?

Most likely it is a combination of psychological and social factors. A man in his middle years often will feel dissatisfied with his achievements in life, will see the world slipping by him. His attainments may not meet his goals; he may feel a bit helpless as his children grow up and are no longer under his control; his job may not be secure.

Under the pressure of acknowledging what he has accomplished in reality, and which of his dreams will remain unfulfilled, a man may doubt his own manhood, his own virility, his own sexuality. As a result he may develop varying degrees of impotence; may be depressed, irritable, nervous, and upset. Thus the male menopause, if we may call it that, is a general physical, psychological, and sexual decline, a combination of aging plus emotional factors.

Is there any cure?

If a man suffers from physical ailments in addition to social and emotional dissatisfactions, good medical care can of course make him more comfortable and self-confident. But chiefly, relief will come only when a man realizes and accepts his limitations. There is no true rejuvenation in seeking a young sexual partner or in male sex hormones. Only a realistic view of life and adjustment in philosophical outlook will bring contentment and serenity.

12. Sex in the Elderly Man

> "Doctor Roen, I've come to see you today not because I'm ill, but because I am in a quandary which requires your medical advice. I am now seventy-one; my wife died five years ago and I'm thinking of marrying again—a woman twenty years younger than I am. I am seeking mainly companionship, but will I be able to act sexually after so many years of abstinence as a widower?"

Although sexual capacity generally declines with age, desire is seldom entirely extinguished. The misconception that an elderly man has no sexual desires can cause great unhappiness. Too often he is segregated from women in old-age homes and other institutions, and if he *does* show any interest in sex or women, he is often accused of being a "dirty old man." The leering attitude expressed in literature and art—such as in the story of Susanna and the Elders—shows a lack of sensitivity to his needs.

Doesn't age reduce a man's physical abilities?

Although the sexual organs do become less active with age, testosterone continues to be produced at such adequate and even high levels that nature obviously expects sexual ability to persist.

Older people would be far better off if their sexuality were viewed realistically: as Freud showed, a man's sexual drive is only partly physical; it is not confined to sexual organs but is largely a behavior pattern, conditioned during earlier years. So it does not disappear at any given age. True, an older man may not be aroused as quickly or as often as in his youth, his erections may weaken, orgasm may take longer—nevertheless these capacities do not vanish simply because he is older.

But don't many older men lose interest in sex?

The persistence of sexual abilities depends greatly on how a man has viewed sex from adolescence onward. Men who have developed a negative attitude, taking part with distaste or aversion, will welcome aging as an excuse to give up sex. A man who has bickered all his married life with his wife gratefully frees himself from a lifetime of poor marital relations by blaming his age. So it is easy to see why one man will be impotent at sixty and another sexually active at eighty.

Then why do so many older men lead sexless lives?

The availability of a sexual partner is crucial. A man whose wife is still living has sexual intercourse more frequently than does an older bachelor or widower. Although the boredom of habit and togetherness discourages sensuality in some marriages, in most instances married life encourages physical contact and arousal. It is easier for the older man living with a woman to continue his sexual activity than it is for the loner with less opportunity for stimulation who must make more of an effort to find a partner.

Then, too, the older married man can often rely on his wife's understanding; chances are their relationship has included previous periods of tension and temporary impotence, and a mutual sharing of faults and frailties; he is therefore not anxious, knowing he will not be criticized should he fail to have or sustain an erection. A bachelor or widower is not as uninhibited—he feels he has to prove his abilities with a new partner, and fears ridicule should he fail.

But don't many older couples also give up sex?

The monotony of many years of marriage can eliminate desire. A man may (even without acknowledging it to himself) have grown tired of his sexual partner because she has aged or for some other reason is no longer alluring. He may even become impotent. When circumstances permit, such a man may almost miraculously regain his vigor by finding a new and physically more attractive mate.

What about widowers?

Loss of a wife may destroy a man sexually, either temporarily or permanently. This may happen because he feels loyalty to his deceased mate or he feels guilty about trying a new sexual encounter, but perhaps even more because of social pressure.

Why do older men give up so easily?

Regrettably, society regards elderly sexual attempts as comic and laughable. Many men simply cannot face this type of ridicule.

What can an older man do, then?

Some men solve this dilemma by turning to prostitutes or other secret liaisons. Others will form an arrangement with a younger woman but often bolster their self-image by giving this woman financial support.

Still others find an answer in masturbation—many men prefer sexual fantasy to an elderly, physically altered wife. One eighty-seven-year-old patient told me about watching an old movie on television that starred an actress he had always liked. That night, he "took her to bed" with him very satisfactorily, and even had an orgasm. What made him proudest, he said, was discovering that after some twenty-five years of no coitus at all, he "still had the power to perform."

Is there any truth to the "dirty old man" stereotype?

Even when the aged male is capable of intercourse, he may also desire less direct forms of erotic satisfaction —these might be pornographic stories, books, or pictures; the company of young women; or indulging in various new sexual experiences such as voyeurism.

Is it true that physically active men retain sexual vigor longer?

It is a general impression that earthy men, such as peasants who have performed hard physical labor during all of their lives, do better and continue longer in sexual activity than those in sedentary occupations. This is not strictly so, for then the same principle should apply to members of the upper classes who also remain physically active throughout their lives through, say, tennis or swimming.

A more valid explanation is that of social inhibiting force, of mores generally related to class hierarchy. The lower-class individual, often less well educated and less inhibited, will be closer to natural urges and drives. The middle-class individual, perhaps "brainier," will be more constrained, introspective, and influenced by many factors and attitudes growing out of his upbringing. Thus this kind of man will be less sexually vigorous only because of the many features already built into him as a result of social ideas and attitudes.

Is it wrong for an older man to be attracted by younger women?

Not at all. Many older men are particularly attracted by younger women. Aristotle Onassis married Jacqueline Kennedy, a woman decades his junior. Pablo Casals at eighty married one of his pupils, aged twenty. Pablo Picasso fathered two children when he was beyond sixty and married still another woman many years later. Charlie Chaplin married young Oona O'Neill when he was many years beyond his "prime" and has had several children with her. These are but a few illustrations that a man is not necessarily finished with sexuality even if his birth date might make people think he is a has-been.

If a man's sexual activities have been pleasant and satisfactory, he will want to continue them into old age. Sex need never die as long as a man lives.

13. Prostaglandins

> "Doctor, while lying here in bed after my own prostate operation, I read in the newspaper that some drug found in a man's prostate is going to help women! How is that possible?"

Prostaglandins, hormones first discovered in male semen, promise to be of enormous importance to *both* sexes.

What are prostaglandins?

Some four decades ago, researchers at Columbia Medical Center found that a component of human semen could contract a woman's uterus. Then Swedish investigators narrowed the active materials down to some chemical compounds that they mistakenly thought originated in the prostate gland and so named these *prostaglandins.*

Now we know that prostaglandins are actually hormones and that they are not confined to the prostate. In fact, they are not even confined to men. Although the highest concentrations *are* in semen—a fact which suggests they are important in reproduction—they are also formed in lesser concentrations in many tissues of the male and female bodies. Yet the term prostaglandins is now so widespread in the medical literature that it is too late to change it.

Why are prostaglandins important to women?

Unfortunately, research in this field is still so new and experimental that so far we have very few answers.

Some components of the prostaglandins, able to stimulate the pregnant uterus, can induce labor with no complications or side effects to either mother or baby. However, we do not yet know whether they offer any advantages over other substances used for the same purpose.

Prostaglandins are also promising for abortion. Given by injection directly into the blood stream of women with early pregnancies in Sweden, Great Britain, and Uganda, they have secured safe abortion in 94 to 100 percent of the cases. These women aborted with only an injection—without instruments, "scraping," intrauterine manipulation, or suction.

In more recent experiments, prostaglandins—painlessly and simply introduced into the vagina by the woman herself—also successfully and safely ended pregnancy. So perhaps in the future a woman might use a vaginal prostaglandin—some sort of medicated tampon—as a method of birth control.

A large American pharmaceutical company has already filed an application for permission to market a prostaglandin drug that terminates pregnancies in the early months.

Why are prostaglandins important to men?

For men, prostaglandins seem to have a special meaning: One study showed that the semen of infertile males contained very low prostaglandin levels compared to a group of normally fertile males. So it is possible that a man's ability to father a child may depend upon his body's ability to produce prostaglandins. If so, couples unable to conceive may be helped by administration of these hormones.

What else can prostaglandins do?

Since prostaglandins have been found to reduce the formation of stomach acids, in both men and women they might help heal and control stomach ulcers.

Prostaglandins have been found to affect blood pressure, and their experimental use on men and women suffering from high blood pressure is promising.

Encouraging experiments are also going on in the use of these chemicals for arthritis.

These are only a few of the potential uses suggested for prostaglandins. Ironically, although prostaglandins were discovered originally in male semen, their specific male genital role seems limited. They may turn out to be more useful for women's reproduction processes and in general medical care.

14. Venereal Disease

> "Doctor, I have a discharge from my penis, and I'm afraid I may have VD. If I do, I must have picked it up from a toilet seat."

The old story that venereal disease can be picked up from a toilet seat is nonsense. Except under unusual circumstances—as in the case of medical personnel working in laboratories or handling infected patients—all venereal disease is transmitted sexually. These germs are simply too fragile to survive on a toilet seat or anywhere else outside the human body.

What are venereal diseases?

These are a group of five communicable maladies whose only common feature is that they are acquired by sexual contact: syphilis and gonorrhea are the most frequent; equally serious but rarer are chancroid, granuloma inguinale, and lymphogranuloma venereum. The germs or organisms that cause these diseases are completely different from each other, and one cannot change into another. It is, however, possible for a person to have more than one at the same time.

Although modern drugs had caused a steady decline in these infections for over twenty years, recently the diseases have been making a comeback. Today there is almost an epidemic, especially of gonorrhea. This upsurge is very likely related to better birth-control methods (especially the Pill) and a change in moral and social attitudes that has encouraged greater sexual freedom.

What are the symptoms of gonorrhea?

The mucous membrane or lining of the urethra is very susceptible to invasion by the gonococcus which causes this disease, and about two to ten days after the sexual contact that infected him, a man will suddenly have burning on voiding and notice a thick, creamy discharge. Only rarely is the discharge so mild a man does not notice it.

The infection may be carried to the eyes and—especially in homosexuals who practice pederasty, or in women—to the rectum.

How is it diagnosed?

The discharge must be examined under the microscope, where the germs are seen as coffee-bean shapes in pairs. Sometimes these bacteria are difficult to identify in the discharge and have to be cultured in laboratory test tubes before a definitive diagnosis is possible.

Can gonorrhea resemble other urologic diseases?

Yes. Inflammations in the prostate (see Chapter 2), kidney diseases, and nonvenereal infections in the urethra can also cause burning on urination and even a whitish discharge.

Sometimes, as with infections caused by the trichomonas bacteria, microscopic analysis will differentiate the cause from gonorrhea. But one common type of urethral inflammation called "nonspecific urethritis" and generally based on a prostatitis is particularly confusing; here microscopic examination of the discharge fails to reveal specific germs, hence the name "nonspecific."

However, the discharge in gonorrhea is typically plentiful, thick, white, and creamy; whereas with nongonorrheal urethritis it is scanty and thin, more watery, resembling mucus (the material you blow from your nose).

Can a man be unaware he has gonorrhea?

Usually not. Most men will notice the discharge and burning on urination. It is therefore unlikely that a man would be an unknowing carrier of this infection.

Is it true that a woman could unknowingly infect a man?

Most definitely. Women are often unknowing carriers of gonorrhea because this disease causes few if any symptoms in them. The germs can travel up the uterus to attack the fallopian tubes and ovaries, so that a woman may become sterile.

In addition, even if a woman does suspect she could have gonorrhea, diagnosis is much more difficult and uncertain than in a man. In fact, sometimes the only way to find out that a woman has the disease is by having her male sex partner acquire it and to diagnose it in him!

Finally, even when a woman has been diagnosed and treated, cure is more difficult than in a man. The reason is that the deep recesses and folds of the vagina provide an ideal environment for these germs, making them inaccessible to antibiotics and likely to survive treatment. Women must therefore be given a high dosage of medication and return more than once for a checkup on the effectiveness of treatment.

How is gonorrhea treated?

A large single dose of penicillin, injected into the buttock, is often curative. Sometimes follow-up injections or oral medications are also given. People who are allergic to penicillin can be given tetracycline or oxytetracycline, both of which are effective.

As some strains of gonorrhea are sometimes resistant

to penicillin, men should always return for a checkup to be certain the cure has worked. Resistant cases can then be treated with other antibiotics.

A man being treated for gonorrhea is usually given a blood test to be sure he doesn't also have syphilis.

What happens if you don't go for treatment?

When gonorrhea goes untreated, or when the gonococci prove resistant, the germs may extend deeper into the urinary tract, to the prostate and neck of the bladder. Urgency and frequency of urination result, and occasionally voiding of blood.

Prostatic abscesses may form, or the man may develop epididymitis, which often results in sterility. Another serious but fortunately rare complication is gonococcal arthritis: a joint such as a knee swells with pus and becomes painful. Gonococcal infections of the heart or brain (meningitis) are even more uncommon but can occur when the disease is untreated.

What is syphilis?

This disease, totally different from gonorrhea and potentially much more serious, is caused by a microbe called a spirochete, which can be seen only by a special microscopic technique (dark-field examination). The microbe, which is thin and shaped like a spiral, is easily destroyed by drying, or by exposure to sunlight or disinfectants. It is spread by intimate contact, either genital or oral.

What are the symptoms?

There are three stages of syphilis, and each stage has its own symptoms:

In the early or *primary* stage, a sore (chancre) appears—generally on the penis or lip—usually about ten days to three weeks after sexual exposure. The lymph glands adjacent to this sore swell and become slightly tender. Even without treatment the sore heals, usually without any scar, but the disease remains in the body.

In the second stage, called *secondary syphilis,* the spirochete travels through the blood stream and multiplies throughout the body—especially in the skin, the eyes, the nervous system, and the mucous linings. About six weeks after the initial infection, there is a skin rash, slight fever, persistent sore throat, eye inflammation, and some evidence of nerve attack. Many ailments may be simulated by this secondary syphilis, which has been called the "great imitator." Any or all of these symptoms may exist from a few days to several months and then disappear. A *latent* phase of syphilis may now follow, lasting from a few months to many years, during which there is no outward sign of the disease.

Late syphilis comes on after an uncertain time. It can take different forms, among which are cardiovascular syphilis (heart and blood-vessel involvement) and neurosyphilis (brain and spinal-cord disease), both of which are very grave and disabling and lead to death.

How is syphilis diagnosed?

Usually with a blood test. However, a blood test on someone who has just contracted syphilis is often negative; it may take from a few days to one or two weeks for a blood test to be positive.

How is syphilis treated?

The most effective remedy for syphilis is penicillin in large doses. It is, of course, ideally treated in the primary stage. In later stages, any damage inflicted by the disease remains and is not reversible; treatment then simply halts further destruction.

Syphilis can be passed on to an unborn child by an infected mother. This congenital syphilis in the child has its own signs and is easily recognizable, but it is fortunately rare now in more advanced countries because of routine and mandatory blood testing of all pregnant women.

What about the other three venereal diseases?

Chancroid, granuloma inguinale, and lymphogranuloma venereum are far less common than gonorrhea and syphilis. Each is characterized in the early stages by sores or lesions in the genital or groin areas and by swelling of the lymph glands.

These infections can be diagnosed only through laboratory and tissue tests, and usually a blood test for syphilis is also done. All are treated with antibiotics or sulfa drugs, but complications sometimes require surgery.

15. Vasectomy

Often patients who ask me about vasectomy—because their wives can't tolerate the Pill or they feel that birth control is a man's responsibility as well as a woman's—are not worried about the operation itself. Usually they understand that this is simple and safe. What bothers them, no matter how intelligent or well educated they are, are prevalent misconceptions, such as that they might not be able to have adequate erections, ejaculations, or even a climax.

I am firmly convinced of the need for birth control. The world's population is in a runaway state—exceeding the ability of the planet to house and feed the people of the future. Even if the population growth rate remains constant (at a 2 percent increase each year), 7.5 billion people will be living on earth in the year 2000. Given this growth rate, most countries are expected to experience famines in the 1980's, and the United States before 1990. Food experts predict that the U.S. will no longer have grain to export to under-developed nations within five years; and that by 1980 most foods, including beef and fresh vegetables, will be priced beyond the reach of all but the wealthy. Perhaps housewives, watching the steady rise of prices in their supermarkets, are way ahead of their husbands in realizing how desperately we need birth control.

What is vasectomy?

Vasectomy is an ideal contraceptive—the most reliable method of birth control known today. Safe, easy, and free of side effects, it is a permanent method of ending a man's fertility—in short, it is male sterilization.

What is male sterilization?

Sterilization, which many people unfortunately equate with diminished sexual capacity or even with castration, is nothing of the sort. It is simply a method of terminating a man's ability to impregnate a woman. Vasectomy does this by preventing the sperm from getting into the semen.

How is this possible?

In the illustration of the male genital tract on page 21, you can see that the long thin tubes called the vas deferens run from the testicles to the beginning of the urethra (just where the urethra and the bladder join). Vasectomy (*vas* from the vas deferens, plus *ectomy,* to cut) consists simply of snipping through both of the vas deferens and closing off the cut ends.

This minor surgical procedure prevents the sperm from reaching the urethra, from which point they would normally be ejaculated. A man still has an ejaculation, but it no longer contains sperm.

What happens to the sperm cells?

The testicles stop manufacturing them. However, the testicles retain the *ability* to make sperm; should the ends of the vas deferens be reunited, sperm cells will again be produced and ejaculated. (However, it is difficult to rejoin these ends, and vasectomy should be considered a permanent operation.)

How does vasectomy differ from castration?

Castration is the removal of both testicles. Vasectomy does not damage the testicles or their ability to produce male hormone.

How is vasectomy done?

After an injection of anesthetic into the skin of the scrotum, the doctor makes an incision about one-half to one inch long. The firm tube of the vas deferens can be felt through this incision, and the surgeon will pull

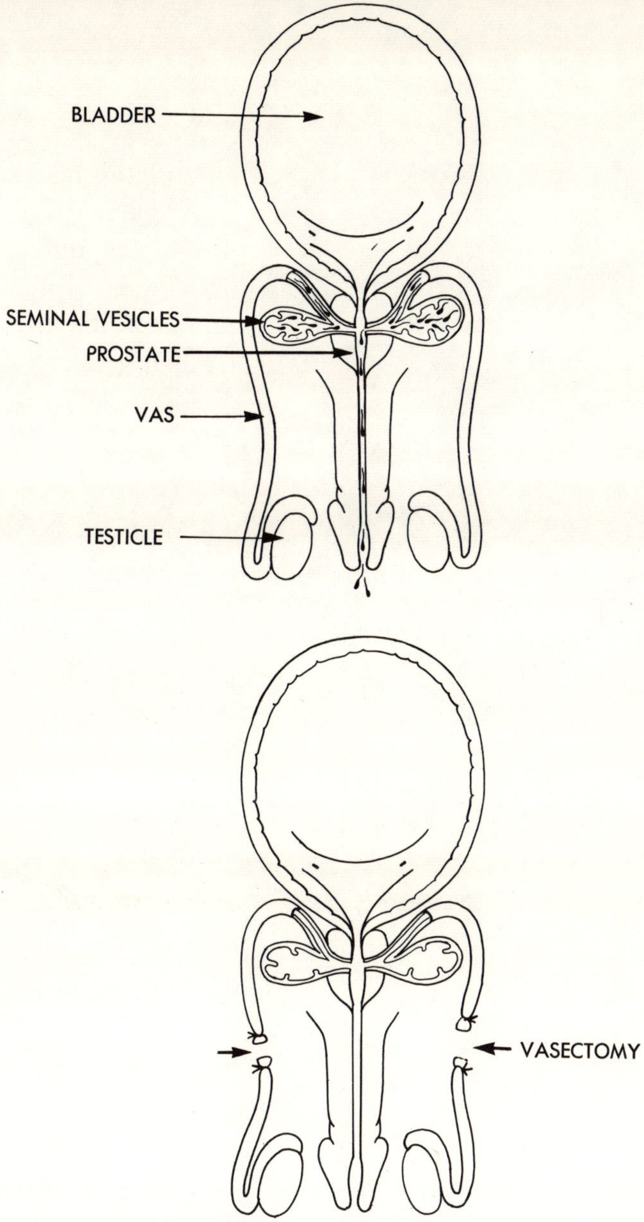

Vasectomy: In vasectomy, the vas deferens is cut and tied off so that the sperm are no longer able to reach the semen. Semen and male hormones are, however, still produced, so that a man's sex life is not affected.

it up gently with an instrument and separate it from its surrounding sheath. Enough of the vas is freed so that the surgeon can cut away about half an inch of the tube. He then ties off the ends of the cut tube, leaving this half-inch gap between them. The gap makes it impossible for nature to bridge the distance; if the ends were too close together, nature, which is so good at repair, might reestablish a connection.

The doctor then stitches the edges of the incision in the scrotum together with a material (catgut) that is absorbed by the body; thus the stitches do not have to be removed later.

Does vasectomy require hospitalization?

Usually not—it is so simple and safe that it is almost always done in the doctor's office under local anesthesia. It takes only fifteen to twenty-five minutes.

Only on the rare individual who is allergic to local anesthesia, or who has a diabetic, cardiac, or other problem, may the physician wish to operate in a hospital under general anesthesia.

Is vasectomy painful?

The surgery is painless because of the anesthetic. Even when the anesthetic wears off, there is no real pain—only a temporary aching, as you might feel from a sore muscle or bruised hand. A vasectomized man can resume his usual physical activities the day after his operation.

Does the operation ever fail?

Occasionally an inexperienced doctor *might* fail to recognize the vas deferens and tie off another tube instead! This has been known to happen, but of course not very often. It is even rarer for nature to reunite the cut tube ends if the vas deferens has been properly cut and tied.

Why do you sometimes hear that vasectomy did fail?

Some men fail to observe one important caution: that they are not *immediately* "safe" or infertile after the operation. This is because sperm cells that were produced prior to the vasectomy are still stored in a man's genital system—and the only way to get rid of them is through ejaculation. It generally takes half a dozen orgasms to expel them, and for this period the couple must use their customary contraceptives.

After several emptying ejaculations, the doctor must examine a semen specimen under the microscope to determine whether any sperm cells are left. Only when sperm are no longer seen in the ejaculated fluid is the vasectomized man "safe."

Does vasectomy affect male hormones?

No. After vasectomy the testicles keep on making testosterone (male sex hormone) in the same quantity and quality as before. Moreover, since testosterone (unlike sperm) does not travel via the vas deferens but is absorbed into the blood stream, its absorption is not affected. Thus vasectomy does not alter any male characteristics.

Does a man feel different after vasectomy?

My experience, after having performed innumerable vasectomies, is that this operation will not change your sexual ability, libido, or sexual needs. The mere tying off of a sexual duct does not affect your hormone production, nerves, or sexual organs. Seminal fluid is produced and ejaculated as usual, so there is no difference in orgasm or climax.

Nor does the man who has had a vasectomy feel physically or emotionally different—though some men say that the relief at not worrying about pregnancy makes them feel a whole lot better!

The only difference is invisible—your ejaculate no longer contains sperm. But this is hardly anything a couple is going to notice, since it can be verified only with a microscope.

Does vasectomy improve your sex life?

Many men—and their wives—find that vasectomy eliminates emotional stress accompanying sex because it removes fear of an unwanted pregnancy.

In an interesting study of 1,012 vasectomized men conducted by the Simon Population Trust (which runs a vasectomy clinic in Cambridge, England), 73.1 percent said their sex life had improved, 25.4 percent said it had not changed at all, and only 1.5 percent said that their sex lives were less satisfactory. When the wives of these men were interviewed, 79.4 percent of these women said their sex lives had improved, for 20.1 percent it remained the same, and for only 0.5 percent had it deteriorated. In addition, 99.4 percent of the men said they had no regrets, and 99 percent said they would recommend the operation to others.

Numerous other studies in the United States and other countries also show that vasectomy improves the emotional state of both members of the couple.

When improvement in sexual ability occurs following vasectomy, it is very likely psychological—the couple is probably more spontaneous and less restrained, and the woman is more willing, because undesired pregnancy is no longer a threat.

What about the 1.5 percent of men and 0.5 percent of women in the Simon Population Trust study who claimed that their sex lives had deteriorated?

Most likely a less satisfactory sex life had nothing to do with the vasectomy but resulted from other physical changes which had occurred in the couples after the operation—illness in one of the partners, for instance.

Can vasectomy make you ill?

No. Some scare stories—perhaps circulated maliciously by people antagonistic to vasectomy, or innocently by people who don't understand what the operation involves—claim that vasectomy causes multiple sclerosis, arthritis, and a host of other illnesses. These rumors are of course preposterous—none of these illnesses could possibly be linked to the tying off of the vas deferens.

Another fiction is that vasectomy gives rise to harmful sperm antibodies. Again, there is no scientific basis to the story. It is simply that garbled accounts tend to arise around any new procedure before people learn to understand and accept it.

Can vasectomy improve your health?

Men sometimes do claim their general well-being has improved following vasectomy. However, cutting the vas deferens can't improve your health any more than it can damage it. Probably these men just feel better because they are less tense about sex.

Is vasectomy legal?

A good many people, including some misinformed physicians, think that there is something underhanded or illegal about vasectomy. They fear it must be clandestinely performed and are sometimes reluctant about this operation. Such ideas are totally fallacious.

Vasectomy, on a voluntary basis, is legal in all fifty states of the U.S.

In forty-four states, there are no legal restrictions whatever.

In Colorado, Georgia, North Carolina, Tennessee,

and Virginia one or more of the following limitations may apply: 1) medical consultation may be necessary; 2) the operation may not be performed in a doctor's office but only in a hospital; 3) minors must have a compliant court order.

In Utah, vasectomy is presently allowable only for "medical necessity"—which presumably is interpreted to mean that it is limited to men who might father children with birth defects. But there is a possibility that Utah's law may be declared unconstitutional.

What about religion and vasectomy?

The stands taken by the various religious bodies differ considerably.

The Roman Catholic Church holds that any method of contraception (other than "rhythm"—abstaining from coitus during a woman's fertile period) is morally impermissible. Sterilization is included in this ban. The Roman Catholic thesis is that coitus is for reproduction and that any attempt to alter this is sinful. Although this may act as a deterrent to many Catholics, it is disregarded by many others; the *National Catholic Reporter* published the following statistics on six hundred men undergoing vasectomy at the Midwest Population Center in Chicago: 44 percent were Protestant, 39 percent were Roman Catholic, 3.7 percent were Jewish, 1.4 percent were not affiliated with any religious group, and 11.9 percent did not state their religion.

Most other organized religious groups or churches do not have any official stand, preferring to leave decisions on intimate matters up to the individual. Nevertheless, many prominent theologians and clergymen of various persuasions have endorsed vasectomy. One such leader is Bishop John Wesley Lord of the Methodist Church, who has said: "I personally believe that voluntary sterilization, practiced in Christian conscience, fulfills rather than violates the will of God."

What if you change your mind?

Although I approve of vasectomy, I always counsel my patients that this operation is permanent and *not* reversible.

Theoretically it *is* possible to operate again and reconnect the cut ends of the vas deferens. But in practice, the chances of successfully reconnecting them are very low indeed—less than 5 percent. Even if a surgeon reconstructs the vas deferens so that sperm reappears in the ejaculate, the number of sperm cells is so low that pregnancy seldom occurs. This is not because sperm are not being produced by the testicles but because the reconstructed vas deferens loses its efficiency in carrying them to the urethra. I therefore recommend this operation only to a man who is quite certain he doesn't want any more children.

What about sperm banks?

If a couple wants vasectomy, yet fears that in the future their family situation might change and they might want to have children, it is possible to use a sperm bank. Before vasectomy, the man can masturbate and deposit sperm in special receptacles. These specimens are frozen and stored at temperatures low enough to keep them immobile but alive. Should the couple decide they want another child, these preserved sperm cells can be used in artificial insemination of the wife to produce a successful pregnancy. So it is possible for a man to father a child in this way even years after vasectomy.

On a broader horizon, sperm banks give rise to intriguing thoughts of preserving sperm cells of superintelligent men or men of special characteristics to impregnate women years, decades, or perhaps even centuries after the death of the donors.

Index